You Can Beat the Odds on Heart Attack

You Can Beat The Odds on Heart Attack

by Irving M. Levitas, M.D.
with Libby Machal

The Bobbs-Merrill Company, Inc.
Indianapolis / New York

Contents

FOREWORD

There is a diminishing number of "purists" who feel justified in saying, "Until it is *proven* that we can prevent atherosclerosis and its complications, such as coronary heart disease, don't worry the population or individuals about unproven changes in diet, habits and life style." Dr. Irving Levitas has taken the other tack in this encouraging book that views Coronary Risk Factor reduction as a prudent policy and presents specific guidelines for an individualized approach. Not all medical scientists will agree with all specific recommendations, but I believe there will be few practitioners who won't welcome a patient's inquiry about his or her specific status and possible program after reading this thoughtful review.

The text is readable and straightforward, with an avoidance of medical jargon. We are not subjected to a collection of anecdotes which suggest but clearly do not prove benefits resulting from certain actions. Dr. Levitas could give us many such encouraging notes from his extensive clinical experience, and particularly from his widely recognized and successful rehabilitation program for heart attack patients. As a leader in this field, he has kept up with the literature from Canada and the United States and from many other countries, and yet, he has not overwhelmed us with minor points.

It is particularly helpful that he has been so explicit in providing guidelines for a program of increased physical activity, an aspect of medical practice that has yet to be adequately covered in the curriculum of most medical schools. His experience with exercise testing and training has given him a middle-of-the-road approach that avoids the hazards of those espousing competitive running or the discouragement of those who fear to take even minimal chances.

That risk factor reduction will be firmly proven of preventive value will take another five, ten or even more years under the present research program of this and other countries. In the meantime, Irv Levitas and I and many other physicians believe we can help our patients if we can persuasively motivate them toward a healthier life style.

This book should help many to prevent disease and, along the way, find enhanced health and an improved quality of life.

Samuel M. Fox 3rd, M.D.

The Day of a Heart Attack –
One Man's Experience

I'LL CALL HIM MONTE. He was the vice president of a company that imported and sold souvenirs. On that morning, as on most mornings, he awoke at six o'clock, half an hour before the alarm was to go off, his brain already wrestling with the office problems that lay ahead. The union wanted another raise; he was to meet with the union representatives over lunch. Before that he had to track down a shipment of souvenirs delayed in Marseilles. He would put off all other business until the afternoon, then return calls and dictate answers to the pile of mail—or maybe take the mail home and work on it in the evening.

He organized his day as he dressed, going over and over the details in his mind. He brushed his teeth carefully, returned the tube of toothpaste to the medicine cabinet, then paused for a moment, examining the cabinet's contents. He felt the beginning of a headache, no more than a heavy pulse in his temple. Perhaps he could stop it before it grew into the throbbing pain that bothered him frequently of late. He made a mental note to call his doctor for an examination—he'd skipped the last two annual check-ups because the doctor always told him he was in good health. He opened a bottle of aspirin and spilled two tablets into his palm. From a smaller vial he added a Valium, a tranquilizer originally prescribed for his wife, Joan, but now shared by both of them. He washed down the three pills with a swallow of water from his cupped palms, returned the aspirin to its place in the cabinet and slipped the Valium into his trousers pocket. He might need it later.

The children, both in high school, were still asleep when Monte came downstairs. But Joan was already up and about, starting breakfast. The conversation had become something of a ritual.

"Good morning, hon."

"Morning."

"Sleep well?"

"Fine. You?"

"Fine. How many eggs?"

"Two, please."

Monte liked a big breakfast. This morning he would eat two eggs over light, four slices of bacon, orange juice, two slices of buttered toast with jam, coffee with cream and sugar. Although Monte weighed 20 pounds more than in his Army days during the Korean War, the extra pounds didn't show much on his muscular, broad-shouldered frame. If he were a little thicker through the middle than he used to be, he could console himself with the observable fact that he still looked to be in better shape than most other forty-four-year-olds he knew. Anyway, he'd already promised himself to take up tennis as soon as the weather turned milder. He'd played handball in his younger days, before office responsibilities took up so much of his time and before he moved out of the city. No one seemed to play handball much in the suburbs. And let's face it, that's a tiring sport. A man his age had to take things a little easier.

Over breakfast Monte glanced at the news summary on the front page of the *Wall Street Journal,* then turned to the stock tables. The market was down again. Once more he felt that familiar warning pulse in his temple and decided against checking his stocks. He asked Joan for another cup of coffee, opened a fresh package of Parliaments, lit a cigarette and inhaled deeply, with satisfaction. That first cigarette in the morning was always the best, he thought, better than any of the twenty to thirty other cigarettes he would smoke as the day wore on.

The first cigarette squashed out and a second lit, Monte kissed Joan on the cheek, struggled into his coat, picked up his attaché case, and walked to the garage. He buckled the seat belt and shoulder strap carefully for the forty-minute drive to town. He'd seen a lot of ugly accidents in the seven years he'd been commuting. All the statistics clearly indicated that he was much more likely to survive a bad crash if he buckled up. Taking precautions against a car accident was just plain common sense.

He arrived at the office at eight-thirty. The others would start straggling in at nine. Then the phones would start, too. Meanwhile, he had half an hour of quiet to review the papers in his attaché case and organize the morning's work for Miss Baron, his secretary. His workday had just begun, yet Monte already felt tired, drained of energy.

He blamed the tranquilizer.

Monte was in his shirtsleeves when Miss Baron arrived. By noon, after three hours on the transatlantic phone, his tie was off and he was perspiring heavily, although his office wasn't unduly warm. He asked Miss Baron to order roast beef sandwiches, potato salad, and beer for the meeting scheduled to start in the conference room at twelve-fifteen—and to open the windows. He washed, changed his shirt, and put on his tie and jacket. He liked to look right at meetings.

The meeting went about as he'd expected. The union people lost their tempers and pounded the table. He kept his under control. He'd trained himself to look cool during negotiations. That gave him an edge. Afterward, though, the headache broke through the shield of aspirin. He blamed the beer. Beer always gave him a headache. He usually drank Cokes at lunch.

Monte worked lethargically through the afternoon. His head

still hurt, he was sweating again, and now he had heartburn. He took a DiGel tablet and swore he'd give up lunchtime negotiations. By four-thirty, still feeling full and extremely tired and weak, he decided to beat the rush-hour traffic home and catch up with his work after dinner. He crammed the papers on his desk into the attaché case and asked Miss Baron to leave a message with his wife if anything urgent came up after he left.

Joan was surprised to see her husband pull into the garage at five-fifteen. He rarely made it home before nine. Michael, his twelve-year-old, was delighted. His father had promised to put up the basketball backboard, bought as a Christmas present three months before, first chance he got. Now was the chance, Michael thought.

No soap. "I feel a little under the weather," Monte told his son. "I want to take a nap. This weekend. I promise."

He intended to keep that promise, too. He knew what it was like to need a father. His own father, apparently healthy but for a "mild" case of diabetes, died suddenly when Monte was only eleven. They say he died of excitement. He keeled over while listening to a radio broadcast of the 1941 World Series. Mickey Owens, a catcher for the Brooklyn Dodgers, had just dropped a third strike pitched to Tommy Henrich of the Yankees. Henrich reached first and the Yankees went on to win the game. When Monte's father fell off his chair, the family thought he was joking.

"Should I wait dinner for you?" Joan asked.

"No, no. I'll have the usual, later."

The usual was a sirloin steak, mashed potatoes, and Coca-Cola. Monte ate the same dinner every night, except on the occasional evening when he took the family out. He liked steak and potatoes, and it was a meal Joan could prepare with a minimum of fuss.

Monte climbed the stairs, shedding his coat, jacket, tie, and shirt on the way. He felt oppressed and weak, as if the world were caving in on him. Deciding he needed a sleeping pill, he detoured to the bathroom and headed for the medicine cabinet. Here's how he describes what happened next:

"I felt like someone hit me in the chest with a hot sledge hammer. My arms went numb and began to burn. I fell down and vomited. Then I passed out. When I came to, I was in the hospital with tubes stuck in me."

At the age of forty-four, Monte had his heart attack.

Statistically, he could hardly have missed. Although careful to take precautions against automobile accidents, which kill about 55,000 Americans each year, he took no precautions against a heart attack, the end result of a chronic but usually hidden disease that kills some 750,000 Americans each year. Indeed, he lived a life that seemed to invite a heart attack— not eventually, at the age of sixty-five or seventy, but just then, in the prime of life.

One-third of all heart-attack deaths occur before the age of sixty-five. Men suffer seven out of every ten heart attacks. To put it another way, three men have heart attacks for every woman who has one. The average American male stands one chance in five of suffering a heart attack *before* the age of sixty. That alone is an appalling statistic. Yet, if you change a detail here and there, you'd find Monte's day not very unlike that of millions of men in their middle years. Certain risk factors increase the chance of premature heart attack far beyond the average one in five.

- When a fatty diet loads the blood with fats and cholesterol, the risk of premature heart attack nearly doubles.
- High blood pressure also doubles the average risk.
- A cigarette smoker runs nearly twice the risk of a non-smoker.
- A diabetic's risk of heart attack is two to three times greater than average.
- Obesity forces the heart to work harder and increases the risk.

- Lack of exercise is also closely related to premature heart attacks. It encourages obesity. It leaves the heart unprepared for sudden stress.
- A family history of heart disease makes premature heart attacks more likely.

Most important, a combination of those risk factors multiplies the risk enormously. An overweight man with a high level of fat and cholesterol in his blood, high blood pressure, and a heavy cigarette habit runs more than five times the average risk of premature heart attack. Monte was such a man. His diet led to overweight and undesirable levels of fat and cholesterol in the blood. Pushed by a life of tension, he smoked inordinately. He had developed high blood pressure since he'd last seen his doctor; that, or nervous tension, might have accounted for his frequent headaches. His sedentary habits aggravated all the clinical conditions.

If there were such a thing as a medical bookmaker, he could give you no better than even money, had you wanted to bet that Monte would make it to sixty without a heart attack. And if you wanted to place a more modest bet—merely that Monte would *live* to sixty—you wouldn't get much better odds. About 25 percent of those who suffer their first heart attack die within three hours; another 10 percent die within three weeks. Overweight patients or those in poor physical condition are much less likely to survive a heart attack than those who have stayed in shape.

Had Monte died, his obituary the next day might have mentioned that he'd died of "natural causes." That's one of many common misconceptions about heart disease, the notion that it's natural. It certainly isn't natural in a man of forty-four. It's merely common, the end result of a decidedly unnatural life.

Anthropologists tell us that primitive people lived on a diet of grains, vegetables, fruit, and small animals; in other words, they were omnivorous. Totally herbivorous animals have jaws and teeth adapted to chewing vegetable matter. The jaws of totally carnivorous creatures are adapted to tearing off and chewing raw meat. Humans, however, are halfway between vegetable-eaters and meat-eaters. They don't have a jaw structure that's suitable for dealing with large raw animals. The discovery of fire—a means of tenderizing meat —opened up a whole new gastronomic world to primitive people, who soon learned to enjoy the taste of (cooked) large animals; they also learned to drink milk other than that of their mothers.

Humanity hasn't adapted to those dietary mistakes yet.

Evolution equipped us to roam large areas in search of food. We walked and ran continually to stay alive. Those too old or too ill to hustle either died or lived on the charity of more vigorous kinsmen. But human beings learned to alter that harsh scheme. We have organized a mechanized life of plenty attained with minimum physical effort.

But our bodies rebel at that life.

Our nervous system attuned itself over millions of years to respond to occasional sudden danger. Thus, we react to an emergency with a fast but brief burst of energy, enough to fight an enemy or run for our lives. Physiologically, modern men and women respond to an emergency precisely as primitive people did. But we have learned to suppress, at some cost, our intuitive drive to fight or flee in most emergency situations. Doing neither, we fail to discharge the nervous energy our bodies build up. Our hearts, designed by evolution to cope with occasional emergencies between long periods of tranquility, are asked instead to cope with the constant emergency represented by the high level of stress built into modern industrial society.

The sales figures for tranquilizers and sleeping pills, the most frequently prescribed classes of drugs in this country, show that Americans are trying to cope. The morbidity and mortality figures for heart attacks and strokes indicate that we're failing. Indeed, despite all the medical advances since 1920, the life expectancy of a forty-year-old American male has remained virtually unchanged. Premature heart attacks and strokes have filled the death gap opened by the conquest of so many infectious diseases.

The epidemic of heart disease among young and middle-aged men is a peculiarity of modern industrialized society. (Women have had a better record, but recently they've started catching up to the men.) As we shall see later, in those societies deprived through choice or poverty of foods rich in animal fat, heart disease remains largely a consequence of old age. The same is true where people still walk and run from one place to another; where life still moves at a leisurely pace; where tranquilizers are still unknown and unneeded.

Is it possible to remain a part of modern society and still change your way of life sufficiently to beat the odds on a heart attack? A growing body of evidence now suggests that it is.

2

The Heart Attack—
What It Is and What Causes It

THE HEART ATTACK that finally felled Monte was actually no more than a symptom of a disease that probably began before he was five years old. Not long ago doctors commonly called the ailment "degenerative" heart disease because it is, literally, a degeneration of the arteries of the heart. Now it has a number of names. It's called coronary heart disease in honor of the arteries that encircle the upper part of the heart like a crown, or corona. It's also called atherosclerosis. Since *athere* means "mush" in Greek, atherosclerosis can be loosely translated to mean "mush in the arteries."

That loose translation describes the problem of heart disease rather closely. The inner lining, or *intima*, of a healthy artery is as slick and glistening as polished tile, allowing blood to flow through the artery with little friction. Just as there are small spaces where tiles adjoin one another, there are small spaces between the cells that make up the arterial lining.

Blood flows through the arteries continuously, carrying oxygen and food to all the cells of the body. Given a diet heavy in fat and sugar, or given certain disease conditions, the blood may contain an abnormally high level of fatty particles, some of which are too large for the cells to use. Some of these, in the form of a substance called cholesterol, lodge in the spaces between the cells of the intima, roughening the once-smooth arterial wall and narrowing the passageway through which the blood flows. The trapped fatty substances tend to mass in one or more locations, building into gobs of mushy material called *plaques*. Eventually calcium, also carried in the blood, hardens the plaques.

Atherosclerosis can develop in any artery, but for unknown reasons the mushy deposits appear to attack the coronary arteries sooner than they attack the arteries elsewhere in the body. Plaques may grow in one or more of the small arterial branches leading from the main coronary arteries without developing significantly in the main arteries at all; or atherosclerosis may attack the larger arteries and not the smaller ones.

No matter where the disease develops, however, it eventually impedes the supply of blood to some part of the heart muscle. If no great demands are made upon the heart—if the heart is never asked to work hard as a result of exercise or emotional upset—it may function well enough even with a decreased supply of the vital oxygen carried by the blood.

Usually, however, a lowered oxygen supply will reveal itself in symptoms. Many patients who suffer a heart attack remember afterward having felt unusually fatigued for a month or two before the attack. Prolonged fatigue could indicate interference with the heart's oxygen supply.

Another early sign of impaired oxygen supply is extra heartbeats, or *extrasystoles*. If the heart's pacemaker, a specialized part of the heart that governs the regular beat, fails to receive its normal oxygen supply, other parts of the heart less well suited to the job may initiate the beat. The patient may have the feeling that his heart is skipping beats every few minutes. Or the heart may start to beat rapidly, as if the patient had been exercising. Extrasystoles can result from many causes other than atherosclerosis, including nervous tension. The feeling of extra heartbeats does not necessarily mean a heart attack is impending. But it may mean just that, and therefore it should be reported to a physician.

A severe and extremely dangerous form of abnormal heart rhythm is called *ventricular fibrillation.* That's a condition in which the heart rhythm changes from a coordinated contraction to a kind of shiver—the muscles of the ventricles fibrillate, or tremble without coordination, rather than an effective beat. The action is so weak that the heart pumps little or no blood —the pump just stops pumping. The patient loses consciousness almost immediately, as the oxygen supply to the brain is cut off. Unless the regular beat is restored within a very few minutes, he dies. Sometimes ventricular fibrillation starts and stops spontaneously, accounting for mysterious fainting spells, particularly in older people. Often, however, a normal beat can be restored only by fast and energetic first aid administered by someone trained in cardiac resuscitation.

Another symptom of impaired oxygen supply to the heart is *angina pectoris,* which means "tightness or stricture in the chest." Some people describe angina less as pain than as a squeezing, oppressive feeling directly behind the breastbone, or as a feeling of breathlessness. The pain or squeezing feeling may radiate from the chest into the neck or the shoulders and arms. An angina patient may sometimes feel the pain in the lower part of the chest and attribute it to indigestion.

The pain of angina pectoris lasts only a few minutes. If it lasts longer—thirty minutes, say—it becomes by the magic of medical definition a condition called *coronary insufficiency,* words that merely mean insufficient blood supply through the coronary arteries. The difference between angina pectoris and coronary insufficiency is a matter of degree. Coronary insufficiency is angina pectoris that lingers.

None of the consequences of atherosclerosis mentioned thus far—fatigue, extrasystoles, ventricular fibrillation, angina pectoris, and coronary insufficiency—is strictly speaking a "heart attack," since none causes permanent damage to the heart muscle. That statement of definition, of course, may prove to be of little comfort to the widow of a man who died suddenly as a result of ventricular fibrillation. But it should at least comfort those who suffer from angina or who experience extrasystoles to know that their hearts may be just as good as anyone else's. It's the coronary arteries that need attention. Atherosclerosis has narrowed one or more of them to the point where they cannot deliver large supplies of blood when the heart demands it. Thus the heart experiences *temporary* shortages of oxygen, shortages you feel as fatigue, extra beats, or pain.

Let's say you are playing tennis and feel a tightness or pain in the chest caused (although you may not know it) by a coronary artery's failure to supply oxygen in the large quantities demanded by your rapidly beating heart. If, as would seem sensible, you quit the game and sat down, the pain might soon subside as the heart's workload declined to the point where there was no longer an oxygen deficit. Suppose, however, that you refused to allow a little "indigestion" to force you off the court, especially when it's your service with a five–four lead in the set. You continue to play (badly, in all likelihood) through angina and through the extension of angina called coronary insufficiency, allowing your heart to go far longer than it should with far less oxygen than it needs. The probable result will be what is called a *myocardial infarction*—death of heart muscle tissue.

That's a classical heart attack.

Thus a myocardial infarction, the heart attack, like angina pectoris and like coronary insufficiency, is a result of oxygen starvation. It can occur from a reduced oxygen supply combined with an increased oxygen demand continued over a relatively long period of time.

But a heart attack can also strike when you're resting peacefully, with your heart beating slowly and making no unusual demands for oxygen. Blood pressure tends to fall when you rest. With a lowered blood pressure, not enough blood may get through the narrowed coronary arteries to feed the heart muscle. Such an attack may occur when you sleep; it may occur painlessly. You may awake and go about your business without even realizing you've suffered a heart attack. Roughly 30 percent of all heart attacks are silent—painless. They are particularly dangerous because they can damage the heart muscle just as severely as a painful attack, but the patient, unwarned by pain, fails to seek the medical attention that might help ward off or help him survive a second attack.

Sudden heart attacks, apparently unprovoked by heavy activity, happen also when a coronary artery, instead of being narrowed by atherosclerosis, is blocked entirely.

Let's return to the mush in the arteries. You'll recall that these atherosclerotic deposits roughen the once-smooth wall of the arterial tunnel. That increases the friction of the blood against the arterial wall and slows the flow of blood. Blood tends to clot when its flow is slowed. Blood clots form around and near the mushy plaques, causing further roughening and further slowing of the flow of blood. Eventually the clot may cut off the blood flow completely.

Translated into Greek, that's a *coronary thrombosis*—a blood clot in a coronary artery.

Occasionally a combination of calcified plaque and clotted material will break away from the arterial wall before it has grown large enough to block the tunnel. It will then be carried along the arterial pathway like a log drifting downstream. Eventually this bit of debris may reach another portion of the artery already narrowed by atherosclerotic deposits, or it may be carried into a small arterial branch. There it sticks, acting as a stopper. That is an *embolus*—Greek for "wedge-shaped stopper." When an embolus stops up one of the coronary arteries, you have suffered a *coronary embolism*, and cardiac infarction—the heart attack—follows.

We have seen that atherosclerosis eventually results in one or more dramatic cardiac events. The mushy deposits may narrow a coronary artery, resulting in heart symptoms but not necessarily damage to the heart muscle. It may encourage the growth of clots inside the artery that block the flow of blood

—coronary thrombosis. Or it may set the stage for clotted material to break away and stop up an artery at a distant site —coronary embolism.

The seriousness of the consequent myocardial infarction— death of heart muscle tissue—often depends on where the blockage occurred. If a thrombosis or embolism blocks the flow of blood through one of the major coronary arteries, large areas of the heart muscle may die for lack of oxygen. The pump may then grow so weak that the patient is said to be suffering from heart failure. Often, however, the stoppage occurs in a small arterial branch and only a small area of muscle is damaged. After appropriate medical treatment and rehabilitation, the victim of such a heart attack may recover to a state of health better than that which he or she enjoyed before the heart attack. Such would be the case particularly if, as a result of this most unpleasant experience, the patient changed his or her way of life drastically to guard against the second heart attack.

The changes urged on those recovering from a heart attack are of the same type as those we will urge in this book for men and women who have not yet suffered a heart attack. The victim of a heart attack is known to have atherosclerosis; indeed, that heart attack can be viewed as a severe symptom of that underlying disease. The available evidence suggests that every American should assume that he or she also suffers from atherosclerosis in some form. Prudence then dictates the taking of active steps to combat the disease by eliminating the factors that make a crisis likely. We will discuss those factors in detail in the following chapters.

3

Cholesterol–
"Hardening" of the Arteries

MUSH IN THE ARTERIES is not an inevitable part of the human condition. Indeed, the incidence of atherosclerosis, and consequently of death due to heart attacks, varies widely from country to country. The United States and Finland are the most heart-attack-prone countries in the world. Mortality statistics show that during a given five-year period one out of every fifty middle-aged Americans dies of a heart attack; in Finland, the death rate is considerably higher. By contrast, heart attacks kill only one in two hundred middle-aged Japanese over the same five-year period.

Why is the rate of death due to premature heart attack eight times greater in the United States and Finland than in Japan? We know that the difference in racial background isn't the answer. If it were, Japanese who emigrate to the United States would retain their relative immunity to heart-attack death, as would their children. They don't. As Japanese immigrants and their children become Americanized, as they abandon their way of life for ours, their rate of heart-attack death starts to climb. When Japanese-Americans integrate themselves entirely into the American culture, one in fifty of them dies prematurely of a heart attack, just as one in fifty other Americans do.

All the evidence indicates that the most significant difference between groups as far as heart disease is concerned is cultural, not genetic. And the most significant cultural difference is in eating habits. With few exceptions, a comparison of typical national diets shows that a high rate of atherosclerosis, heart attack, and death goes hand in glove with a diet heavy in saturated fat and cholesterol. As a rule of thumb, a saturated fat is any fat that remains hard at room temperature (68° F.). Thus, milk fat—butter and most cheese—is saturated fat, as is the fat of meat. Unsaturated fats, such as vegetable oils, are liquid at room temperature. Cholesterol is found mainly in egg yolk, shellfish, and such organ meats as liver, kidneys, and sweetbreads.

Monte ate meat two or three times a day, breakfasted on eggs fried in butter and buttered toast, and suffered an early heart attack. His Japanese counterpart probably eats meat infrequently, perhaps two or three times a week rather than two or three times a day, eats fish as a main course much more often, likes boiled rice rather than bread and butter, drinks tea rather than milk, and cooks his food in soya sauce, a soybean derivative, rather than butter or pork fat.

Curiously, man is the only animal who develops early atherosclerosis while eating a normal diet—a fact that has led some scientists to conjecture that what we consider "normal" isn't normal at all.

The recent discovery of the Tasaday tribe in the Philippines provides a glimpse of how man must have lived millions of years ago, before he outsmarted himself. The Tasaday are what anthropologists call a food-gathering community. They eat only what they can gather fresh each day—berries, roots, frogs, fish, small birds, and other animals that they can catch with their own hands. Until recently they knew nothing of agriculture, animal husbandry, or the fairly sophisticated weapons and traps needed to make large animals a regular part of the food supply. Nor had they learned the cooking skills necessary to make the tough flesh of large animals tender enough for blunt human teeth and weak human jaws.

Perhaps unfortunately for them, the Tasaday were discovered by a hunter who liked to wander far afield in search of game. The Tasaday befriended the hunter, who soon taught them to fashion animal traps and to cook the meat of the large animals they caught. Thus overnight the Tasaday made an error that took the rest of mankind millions of years to bumble into: They developed a taste for the meat of large animals— deer and wild pig.

On most days the Tasaday still follow their easygoing food-gathering habits. Their primitive traps don't work reliably, and butchering, cooking, and devouring the catch is a bit of a chore for a tribe that numbers fewer than thirty men, women, and children. So far, pork and venison are only for great feasts.

It will be interesting to see how long it takes the Tasaday to learn, as the rest of us have learned, that you can domesticate a number of good-tasting animals and keep them in herds, where they will reproduce and free their owners of the inconvenience of hunting and trapping. They will no doubt learn that soon. When they do they will have to solve certain other problems that the rest of mankind has solved. For example, the females in the herd will produce more milk than their young can use. We have learned to drink the milk, churn it into butter as a spread and a cooking oil, preserve it as cheese, freeze it into ice cream, and add it to other dishes as a flavoring.

It is no mere coincidence that Finland, which has the highest heart-attack death rate in the world, also leads the world in per-capita consumption of milk and dairy products. Nor is it a coincidence that the United States, which ranks second to Finland in heart-attack death rate, leads the world in per-capita consumption of beef, pork, and eggs. If a natural or man-made disaster forced Finns and Americans to substitute some other source of protein for much of the milk, meat, and eggs they consume in such abundance, the citizens of both countries would no doubt feel sorely put upon. But the incidence of heart attack would drop sharply.

Such a dietary "disaster" befell Norway during the German occupation in World War II. The Norwegians, who like the Finns normally produce and eat large quantities of milk and dairy products and who normally suffer premature heart attacks at a rate higher than average, found themselves short of milk for their own use. The Germans were taking most of the dairy production for their troops. Having no choice, the Norwegians turned to fruit and vegetables. Even as they grumbled about the wartime shortages, the incidence of coronary attacks declined. With the end of the war, the Norwegian diet returned to normal. Norwegians are again among the biggest per-capita consumers of milk. And they're again among the world's leaders in premature coronaries.

The connection between diet and heart disease is easy enough to trace. Saturated fat tends to increase the body's production of cholesterol, the material that the blood deposits on the arterial walls. Cholesterol is not itself a fat. It's a tasteless, odorless, fatty alcohol produced by the liver as an aid in the production of certain hormones. If we ate no saturated fat or cholesterol, the body would continue to produce it—but it would usually produce only what was needed for normal bodily functions. With a diet heavy in saturated fats and cholesterol, an excess amount of the substance enters the bloodstream, and the rate at which cholesterol is deposited on the arterial walls increases. Obviously, *some* foods containing cholesterol should be eaten. The point is not to overdo it.

The relationship between cholesterol and fats (or lipids) in the blood and the likelihood of some kind of coronary problem is quite close. The higher the cholesterol level in the blood, the greater the chance of a heart attack. Measurement of blood cholesterol and lipids is (or should be) a routine part of every physical examination.

No one knows exactly what a normal cholesterol level in a human being is, or what the most desirable level is. Indeed, it may well be that the normal cholesterol level varies from person to person. However, population studies again point to some clues. Researchers have been studying the life and health of the people of Framingham, Massachusetts, for some twenty-two years now, and have come up with the following statistics: Those with a blood-cholesterol level of up to 220 milligrams per 100 cubic centimeters of blood (called 220 milligrams percent for short, or just 220 for even shorter) suffered an extremely small incidence of heart attack. Those with a cholesterol of 240 suffered heart attacks at a rate average for the population as a whole. And those with cholesterol levels higher than 240 suffered heart attacks more often than average.

Some people have concluded from those figures that 240 is the "normal" blood-cholesterol level and have even taken comfort in that figure. But all you can brag about if you learn from your doctor that you have a cholesterol of 240 (and you should certainly ask) is that you are probably developing atherosclerosis at a rate average for an American. Translation: Your chances of a heart attack are much higher than those of most people in the world, much higher than they should be, and much higher than they need be.

But since 240 is an average figure (the average is higher, 250, for fifty-year-old Americans), few doctors consider that level pathological—a sign of illness. Doctors are trained to attack illness, and when confronted with what they consider to be a high cholesterol, something above the 240–250 range, they attack it with a vengeance, using very effective drugs to reduce cholesterol in the blood and urging a strict diet on the patient.

It's instructive to compare the blood-cholesterol levels of Americans with that of people notably free of heart disease. The people of Vilcabamba, a remote Andean village in Ecuador, came to the attention of medical researchers when it was discovered that thirty-eight of the four hundred adults in the village were between seventy-five and one hundred years old and several other Vilcabambans had passed their one hundredth birthday. The researchers did electrocardiogram studies of the twenty oldest villagers. Only two showed any evidence of heart disease. (By contrast, about 95 percent of Americans seventy-five or older suffer from heart disease.) The average cholesterol level among the adult population of Vilcabamba: 160 to 165.

No heart disease has ever been detected among the aborigines who live in the jungle of central West Malaysia. Their diet consists largely of rice supplemented with other cereals, fish, and fruit. A team of British medical researchers recently studied seventy-three aborigine men over the age of twenty-four. Their median cholesterol level: 143.

Is the American's norm of 240 a sign of illness? I think so. It may not be a cause for *medical* intervention, by which I mean drug therapy and the close supervision of a physician, with all the expense that entails. But it is a sign that you are leading the sort of life that makes you a bad heart risk. You need to start changing the way you live.

A good place to start is at the dinner table. It's a good place to start because you will then change not only the way *you* eat but also the way your family eats. In that way you may add years to the lives of your children. Chapter 6 deals in detail with a healthful manner of eating that should help reduce your cholesterol level and still maintain all the food value needed in everyday living.

Notice I say "manner of eating," not "diet." A diet is something people tend to go on *temporarily*, to lose weight or for some other transient reason. No diet is good enough to beat the odds on a heart attack. What's needed is a new manner of eating—a *permanent* change in eating habits.

Since saturated fat and cholesterol increase the rate of atherosclerosis, its severity, and therefore the likelihood of a cardiac incident, the typical American must reduce the amount of saturated fat and cholesterol he or she eats.

We do need a certain amount of fat for energy. But that

should be unsaturated fat—as far as possible. There are two types of unsaturated fat. Monounsaturated fat (peanut oil and olive oil, for example) neither raises nor lowers blood cholesterol levels. That's better than saturated fat, of course. Better still, however, is polyunsaturated fat (safflower oil, corn oil, soybean oil, and cottonseed oil), because it tends to *lower* existing cholesterol levels. (Coconut oil, although it is a vegetable oil, is a saturated fat.) The American Heart Association recommends that the fat in the diet should consist of one-third each of saturated, unsaturated, and polyunsaturated fats. In Chapter 6 I'll discuss in detail what foods you should be eating.

Can changing your eating habits really reduce the risk of heart attack? Let's look at some of the evidence.

Medical researchers long ago showed that they could produce atherosclerosis in rabbits, rats, chickens, and dogs by feeding the animals a diet high in saturated fat and cholesterol. But those early studies merely proved that a high-fat, high-cholesterol diet was awful for rabbits, rats, chickens, and dogs. Later, medical researchers began experimenting with rhesus monkeys. Rhesus monkeys are very like human beings in the way their body metabolism handles various foodstuffs, and they rarely develop atherosclerosis while eating a stock monkey diet. Early experiments showed that with a high-fat diet you could induce atherosclerosis in monkeys, too. But those experiments were criticized because the damaging foods were fed in abnormal ways, such as intravenously.

It remained for Dr. Robert Wissler and a team of medical researchers at the University of Chicago to show that rhesus monkeys fare poorly when eating a normal American table diet with normal monkey table manners. Dr. Wissler fed a group of middle-aged male rhesus monkeys such foods as milk, eggs, roast beef, pork, cheese, butter, sugar, potatoes, carrots, chicken, cereal, fruit, cake, and juice. He fed a second group of monkeys a diet containing many of the same ingredients, but fewer or no eggs, and less cheese, butter, fatty beef, and pork. The second group of monkeys was also permitted less sugar and about 30 percent fewer calories than the monkeys gorging themselves on the typical American diet.

Within two years, Dr. Wissler reported, there were "grossly discernible" atherosclerotic deposits covering about half the interior surface of the aorta, the body's main artery, in most of the animals eating the American diet. Little disease developed in monkeys fed the low-fat, low-sugar diet, and what atherosclerosis did develop in the second group was much less severe than in the first group.

The University of Chicago study indicates, among other things, that monkeys had best steer clear of the American dinner table. But what of us? We have been eating at that table all our lives. Even granting that changing our manner of eating can lower the level of cholesterol *in the blood,* hasn't the damage already been done in the arteries?

Yes, the damage has probably already been done. But the damage needn't grow worse—and there's even evidence to suggest that it can be undone. Atherosclerosis may well be a *reversible* disease, and a new manner of eating may well be the key to reversing it.

That is the conclusion to be drawn from a recent experiment at the University of Iowa School of Medicine. Researchers there put thirty rhesus monkeys on a cholesterol-building diet containing 40 percent egg yolk for seventeen months. Then they performed blood tests and divided the monkeys into three groups matched for blood-cholesterol levels.

The researchers autopsied one group of monkeys to measure the degree of atherosclerosis in the coronary arteries. They found, not unexpectedly, that they had indeed induced atherosclerosis. The cholesterol content of the arteries of the autopsied monkeys was seven times higher than in the arteries of a control group, which had been maintained from the beginning on a low-fat diet.

The question to be answered, however, was whether a

change in diet would now rid diseased arteries of mush. The two remaining groups of experimental monkeys were put on special diets—one on a low-fat diet free of cholesterol, the other on the same diet enriched with corn oil, a polyunsaturated fat that tends to reduce blood-cholesterol levels. After forty months on the special diet, the cholesterol in the arteries of the monkeys in both groups had declined by 65 percent, although they still suffered from considerably more atherosclerosis than did the monkeys in the control group.

In short, the experiment indicates that even after diet-induced atherosclerosis has developed, a change in the manner of eating can make significant improvements in the disease —that atherosclerosis in rhesus monkeys is to a large extent reversible.

Carefully controlled tests such as those at the University of Chicago and the University of Iowa do more than show that monkeys know what's best for themselves. They help confirm the practical results of dietary tests on human beings.

Back in 1957 the New York City Department of Health formed an Anti-Coronary Club and invited some 800 men between the ages of forty and fifty-nine to join. The club members would change their manner of eating: beef, mutton, and pork in no more than four meals a week; a maximum of four eggs a week; no butter, hard cheeses, or ice cream. Those rules were at the heart of what came to be called the Prudent Diet. After six years on the diet, the club members were compared with a group of some 460 men of the same age who had made no change in eating habits.

During that time, the members of the Anti-Coronary Club had suffered heart attacks, or "coronary incidents," at the rate of 339 incidents per 100,000 people per year. The rate among nonmembers studied was 980 per 100,000 per year. In other words, those who stayed on the diet suffered heart attacks only one-third as often as those who made no change in eating habits.

The biggest controlled dietary study comes, appropriately enough, from Finland. Researchers there studied the inmates of two mental hospitals over a period of twelve years. The main difference between the two groups of inmates was in what they ate. Ordinary milk, butter, and hard (or "hydrogenated") margarine was taken off the menu of one hospital. The whole milk was replaced by skim milk fortified with soybean oil, a monounsaturated fat; the butter and margarine were replaced with a "soft" margarine containing a high percentage of poly-unsaturated fat. After six years, the menus of the two hospitals were reversed. The inmates of the first hospital got back their whole milk. The inmates of the second hospital lost theirs.

Here are some results: In hospital A, the death rate among men from coronary heart disease during the six years of low-fat diet was 7.72 per 100,000 person years. The death rate jumped to 12.97 during the six years on the normal diet. In hospital B, the death rate was 7.5 on the low-fat diet, and 15.18 on the regular diet. Pooling the figures from both hospitals, we find that the rate of death from coronary heart disease was 7.61 on the low-fat diet and 14.08 on the normal diet. In sum, men on a normal Finnish diet *died* of heart disease at a rate more than double that of those on a diet low in saturated fats.

Some still say the case connecting saturated fat and choles-terol directly to heart attacks and heart-attack deaths has not been proven beyond all doubt. The evidence, however, is so strong that, as a practicing physician, I would urge every American—man, woman, and child—to change his manner of eating now.

4

Other Important Food Factors – Sugar and Triglycerides

NEW HEALTH IDEAS take time to filter into everyday medical practice and everyday living habits. It has taken a long time for people to learn to be concerned about cholesterol, and not enough people are yet. But most physicians now know that high blood cholesterol is an important risk factor. And now we're beginning to look at other new ideas about heart disease.

Many of the new ideas which I will discuss in this chapter are still being tested. I think a lot of them will turn out to be important to practicing physicians before too long. Right now they're important only to pure scientists. Pure scientists tend not to accept anything fully until they can get good reliable statistics. But doctors in practice aren't pure scientists, we're social scientists. Over the years, every doctor finds methods of treatment that *seem* to work, even though he can't *prove* that they do. Doctors in practice have to be empirical. We tend to let the medical-school researchers worry about why it works, later on. Our primary concern is to make our patients feel better, right now.

Some of the ideas I'm going to discuss in this chapter are still highly controversial. The day will certainly come when they'll be either accepted or discarded, but, meanwhile, some of them are of immediate use, and I believe you have a right to know about them. I'll give you the pros and cons. Then you can decide for yourself which of them—if any—you might want to work into your own life style.

First and most important is the role of sugar in heart disease, a role that may well go far beyond the role of diabetes (or high blood sugar) alone.

Dr. John Yudkin, a British biochemist, professor of nutrition at Queen Elizabeth College, University of London, has done much of the pioneering research in this field. He's convinced that there is a close relationship between the amount of sugar in the diet and the risk of heart attack. No, he doesn't think high sugar consumption is the only cause of heart disease. He recognizes all the other factors we'll be talking about—smoking, hypertension, lack of exercise, diabetes, etc. But he's convinced that too much sugar is an important factor, *if not a primary cause.*

There was a time when sugar was a great luxury, something only the rich could afford. The only sweetener available to the poor was honey, a form of sugar that is chemically different from refined sugar. There are two kinds of sugar: complex sugar is the kind found in natural products, such as fruits and starches; simple sugar is the *refined* sugar you buy in the supermarket. Incidentally, many people believe that brown sugar contains more nutrients than does white sugar, but this idea is a fallacy. Brown sugar owes its color to impurities; it's merely less refined than white sugar. Dr. Yudkin believes that refined sugar causes undesirable metabolic changes. His studies show that a person who uses 4 ounces of refined sugar a day has a five times greater chance of getting a heart attack than one who consumes only 2 1/2 ounces daily.

In pioneer days, the average American consumed a mere 15 pounds of sugar a year. By the end of World War I our consumption was up to 50 pounds. Since then we've virtually doubled our sugar intake, to an average of about 5 ounces of sugar every day, or more than 100 pounds a year. Some of this sugar is visible. We spoon it into our coffee or tea and use it in cooking. Most of the rest is invisible. We have no way of knowing how much sugar food manufacturers are adding to our processed foods. I'm not talking now about such obvious sweet foods as soft drinks, cakes, and ice cream, but about canned vegetables, soups, pickles, and other foods in which you wouldn't normally expect to find sugar. Take a look at the labels on the cans and jars in your own kitchen, and you'll see exactly what I mean—they say sugar is added, but they don't tell you how much.

If sugar is so bad for us, why did it take so long to realize its potential danger? Primarily because we've only recently learned that the body doesn't handle all dietary carbohydrates in the same way. Total carbohydrate intake varies little from one country to another. We ingest about the same amount of carbohydrate we've always eaten, but the *kind* of carbohydrate is different.

We used to eat more grains and potatoes; nowadays it's more sugar.

Dr. Yudkin has a lot to say about the Samburu and Masai tribesmen of East Africa and the tribesmen of Mongolia, all of whom are very active and eat a tremendous amount of saturated animal fat but suffer very little from coronary thrombosis. These people, he points out, consume almost no sugar. On the other hand, the population of the island of St. Helena, just as active, has a fairly low fat intake, but a high sugar intake—and a high rate of heart disease.

Dr. A. M. Cohen has studied Yemenite immigrants to Israel. These people showed a considerable increase in coronary disease after twenty years in Israel. They had been eating very little more fat than they'd consumed in Yemen, but much more sugar. In all other respects their lives were unchanged.

Why is sugar bad? It's the sugar, both refined and unrefined, that causes the triglycerides in the blood to go up. Next question: What are triglycerides? The triglycerides are fatty acids that are combined with glycerine—a normal fatty substance found in the blood. Three different fatty acids join with the glycerine molecule to form the true fats and oils, the same fats and oils you see in your kitchen—chicken and meat fats, butter, margarine, and cooking oils. In short, triglycerides are nothing more nor less than kitchen fat.

When the amount of triglycerides your bloodstream is carrying becomes too high, they are deposited in the blood-vessel walls, causing atherosclerosis. As you know, some kitchen fats are saturated, some are not. It's the saturates that tend to accumulate on the artery walls.

Dr. Margaret J. Albrink of the University of West Virginia wrote, as far back as 1961, that she found more of her patients showed elevated triglycerides than high cholesterol levels. She also found that triglyceride levels rose as the patients got older. She showed that over 80 percent of heart-attack patients have high triglyceride levels.

Dr. Peter Kuo of Rutgers University thinks that anybody who consumes too many carbohydrates is certain to get elevated blood lipids (triglycerides) and cholesterol. He points out that one 4-ounce chocolate bar contains ten teaspoons of sugar and is the equivalent of five or six slices of bread. It's foolish to believe that fat elevation in the blood has to be due only to fat in the diet, he tells us. He prefers to blame much of it on the excessive starches and sugars we consume.

An experiment at Brookhaven National Laboratory alternated diets high in sugar and high in starch with the same group of subjects. The researchers found that the body changes sugar into two to five times more fat than starch in the bloodstream. In other words, 100 calories of bread is less fattening than 100 calories of candy.

We don't all manage sugar the same way. If your doctor wants to test your ability to handle sugar, he'll order a glucose tolerance test. You'll be asked to drink 100 grams of glucose. Blood samples are then taken to find out how high the blood-sugar (glucose) level climbs.

We know that after a few weeks on a sugar-rich diet many people develop an impaired ability to handle sugar. When you eat refined table sugar, it is absorbed very rapidly. The pancreas then secretes a larger-than-normal amount of insulin into the blood in an attempt to metabolize the sugar and keep the blood sugar from getting too high. Insulin works as an agent to change the glucose into fat, which then can be stored for future use. These stored fats are triglycerides.

A number of years ago we actually gave insulin injections to thin people, before they ate. We told them to take a lot of sugar and starch at the meal. They would gain as much as a pound a day on this regime. However, after we stopped the injections the patients' weight went down again to about what it was before.

Many physicians think that the high insulin level also has something to do with the development of diseased blood vessels. This is why doctors tell diabetics to "keep your diabetes under control," as less insulin is then being secreted.

If a patient who has developed diabetes in adult life—what we call an "adult-onset" patient—cuts way down on his starches and sugars, his diabetes may go away without any other treatment.

That's what happened to many Norwegian diabetics during World War II. Perhaps you remember my telling you that the incidence of coronary attacks declined in Norway when the Germans took the dairy production for their troops, forcing the natives to subsist on a diet of fruits and vegetables. That fruit and vegetable diet also resulted in the disappearance of many patients' diabetes, thanks to the occupying Germans, who were consuming all the available sugar as well as the dairy products.

A good deal of work is being done on the relationships of triglycerides to exercise. Researchers are trying to answer the question of whether young athletes are less prone to the risks of coronary heart disease than are more sedentary young people. They are also attempting to find out if athletic activity in youth is any protection against heart disease in middle age. We know that athletes have much lower levels of triglycerides in their blood, because their muscles use the triglycerides for fuel; thus the triglycerides stay down for a few days following prolonged workouts. The consensus is that the athlete is no different from anyone else once he stops being active.

There is a considerable interest in sports medicine, concerning different types of athletes. Generalizations about athletes are dangerous, since there's such a difference in the demands made by the various sports and in the body types of the competing athletes. Football players and wrestlers are usually endomorphs, while athletes involved in track events tend to be ectomorphic. The words "endomorph" and "ectomorph" define the two basic extremes of body structure. The ectomorph, who is slender, usually goes out for track events such as running and jumping; the endomorph, who is heavily built, has a body that's better adapted for contact sports. Track uses extended effort, something not required of football players and wrestlers. We know that football players tend to eat a lot during the training season. In the interim, when they're out of training, they retain the same food habits, but use far less energy. A study of a group of football coaches, all former athletes, showed that as they grow older they have higher levels of cholesterol and triglycerides, and may actually have a higher risk of heart disease.

Many well-qualified people are still not sold on the importance of triglyceride levels, but as more studies are done, more conclusive results will be obtained.

Next we come to coffee, another bone of contention. There are medical articles written both pro and con. Is it bad? My own opinion is that the harm comes from the sugar used in the coffee rather than from the coffee itself. And I have also noticed that people who drink a great deal of coffee are usually tense individuals, and the excess coffee makes them more jittery. I suspect that the tension more than the coffee is what causes their problems.

The use of alcohol and its relationship to heart disease is another controversial subject. The Kaiser Permanente group in California is having a hard time explaining its finding that there seems to be a slightly higher coronary rate among teetotalers.

Dr. Lawrence Gould of Albert Einstein University warns against the use of alcohol by people who already have some heart damage, as the force of the heartbeat seems to weaken with the use of alcohol. It seems safe to say that one or two drinks are okay; moderate doses of alcohol have been recommended for years as a "good sedative" for heart patients. My own opinion about alcohol is that a drink or two may be preferable at times to the use of sedatives or tranquilizers. Alcohol is a better drug; you won't wake up feeling as foggy. Some recent work has shown that in patients who have what we call Type IV hyperlipidemia (a condition we'll be discussing in Chapter 5), alcohol causes the triglycerides to increase considerably. Such people can't safely drink anything containing alcohol. Even one drink is one too many.

Now let's talk about vitamin E. This vitamin was discovered in 1922 by H. M. Evans and K. S. Bishop. They found that if female rats were to reproduce normally, vitamin E must be present in their diet.

Some investigators have made extravagant claims for it which have not been fully substantiated and which have caused other investigators to repudiate it entirely. One of its most enthusiastic boosters is Dr. Wilfrid Shute of Canada. He believes that vitamin E deficiency is linked to cardiovascular death, but he hasn't been able to prove his point to the satisfaction of the majority of scientists. Maybe someday we will find a relationship between vitamin E and heart disease, but at this time the connection is tenuous at best.

I myself tried an experiment with a small group of angina patients. When I tested these men on a bicycle or treadmill, they developed chest pains, and changes could be seen in their cardiograms. I put them on a dosage of 600 milligrams of vitamin E a day. After about four weeks on this medication, these men all told me they'd begun to feel better. When I retested them, I couldn't find any difference in their responses. They still got chest pains with the same pulse rate.

I could say that their improvement was psychological. But I don't say that, because I have no way of knowing for sure. Perhaps vitamin E improved their nutrition in some way that gave them a sense of well being.

Vitamin E has been called "the embarrassing vitamin" because our skepticism may come back to haunt us some day. Those doctors who have been saying it has no value may have to eat their words. That's why some doctors suggest its use, even though they don't have proof of its value.

Let's summarize the vitamin E facts we're reasonably certain about:

- We know that in the paint industry vitamin E is used as an antioxidant. It keeps the oil in the top of the can from getting a scum on it. This scum forms in the presence of oxygen. We can thus assume that vitamin E must have something to do with oxygen metabolism.
- We know that kwashiorkor is a deficiency disease of children. Use of vitamin E is among the treatments used to improve their nutrition.
- We know that some premature infants are born with a form of anemia that can be cured by vitamin E.
- We know that a lot of physicians (but by no means all) are convinced that vitamin E can be very helpful in the alleviation of cramps in the legs and feet.
- We know that a small amount of vitamin E, given daily, seems to hold in check an uncommon disease called porphyria, in which patients suffer severe abdominal pains, vague muscular discomfort, and nervousness. If a specimen of urine turns black when exposed to sunshine, the diagnosis of porphyria is confirmed.
- We know that some physicians, such as Dr. Alton Ochsner,

the founder of the famous Ochsner Clinic in New Orleans, believe that the administration of vitamin E prior to operation prevents blood-clot formation following the surgery.

- We know that dieticians state that 30 milligrams of vitamin E daily is necessary for good nutrition, and if polyunsaturated fats are increased in the diet, more vitamin E is necessary. Surveys show that most people don't ingest that much in their food.

- We *don't* know what side effects might ensue from overdosage because none are known so far. So long as you take your vitamin E in moderate doses, it will probably do you no harm.

It's interesting to note that I have many doctor friends who have heart trouble—and they're taking vitamin E themselves. In other words: If something has no ill effects and seems to work for you, fine. It's a free country!

Many other vitamins have been credited with a wide variety of remedial properties. In the field of vitamin C, some small amount of work has been done. Dr. Constance Spittle from Yorkshire, England, found that she could lower her own cholesterol by dosing herself with vitamin C. I know of no other studies to confirm her original finding.

Another vitamin that may turn out to have a role in atherosclerosis is vitamin D. Some studies indicate that too much vitamin D may increase the amount of cholesterol in the blood. As you know, the milk in this country is fortified with it and babies get it also as supplements. In France the law prohibits the addition of vitamin D to milk, and the incidence of heart disease is fairly low.

Our methods of treating milk are being questioned. Dr. Kurt A. Oster suspects that boiling milk before drinking it, as the French do, may destroy an enzyme in cow's milk that causes fats to stick to the artery walls. He is also convinced that homogenizing milk breaks up the large fat particles into much smaller ones, which are absorbed into the system more rapidly, thus carrying more of this enzyme into the blood. Also, the rapid surge of blood fats creates problems similar to those resulting from a too-rapid surge of blood sugar. Be that as it may, Dr. Oster finds that in countries where milk is boiled and not subjected to homogenization, the incidence of atherosclerosis is much lower. He also points to those Masai tribesmen who ingest large quantities of nonhomogenized milk without ill effects. Proof of this theory will have to wait until some enterprising researcher puts a group of Masai on a homogenized-milk diet.

The finding that there appears to be a lower incidence of atherosclerosis in parts of the world where the water is hard than in soft-water areas has led some investigators to do studies of the role of calcium and other metals in heart disease. Calcium joins with fats to form soaplike substances which then proceed to be excreted through the intestinal tract. A possible explanation is that, in hard-water areas, where there is more calcium in the water, less fat gets into the bloodstream. Also, the different acid content of waters may affect the quantities and kinds of metals dissolved in them. Recently, elements such as lithium, zinc, magnesium, chromium, etc., which are found only in minute quantities in water and food, are being studied. Improper amounts might be toxic to heart muscle.

Some heart patients also show an elevated uric-acid level in their blood. No one is sure just what this means, but it seems a fairly common finding.

All these pros and cons are very confusing, I know. Food chemistry is extremely complex. However, the important thing is that we are beginning to inquire into the relationship of foods to our health. The outlook is optimistic.

5

Blood Typing for Fats— How Important Is Heredity?

TODAY, WHEN YOU CONSULT your doctor, you take for granted that he'll draw some blood. You can be sure he'll test it for cholesterol, and he's likely to test for triglycerides. Then he may take some of that blood, separate the red and white cells from the plasma, and put the plasma in a refrigerator. The following day he'll look at the tube to see if there are fats floating on the top and whether the serum below is clear or cloudy.

You know that when you put freshly made soup into the refrigerator the fat will rise to the top as it cools. Excess fat in your blood will do the same thing. If "the icebox test," plus cholesterol and triglyceride determinations, shows abnormalities, the doctor may say, "We're going to do a further typing to find out what kind of lipoproteins you have."

Let's back up for a moment while I explain what these lipoproteins are. As you know, oil and water don't mix. Lipids—or fats—are insoluble in water; but in the blood they are bound with protein so that they dissolve, forming lipoprotein molecules.

The following lipoproteins can be identified:
• Alpha lipoproteins, which carry most of the phospholipids.
• Beta lipoproteins, which carry most of the cholesterols.
• Prebeta lipoproteins, which carry most of the triglycerides.

The role of the alpha lipoproteins is still obscure in relationship to heart disease, but we know that the beta and prebeta lipoproteins have a great deal to do with it. We now classify them into five types (or six, if you divide Type II into A and B). Type I and Type V are both very rare and seem to have little practical connection with heart disease in the overall picture, but the others do. Of these, the most important are Type II—characterized by high levels of cholesterol, and Type IV—characterized by normal or moderately elevated cholesterol but high triglyceride levels.

Dr. George Christakis, director of the nutrition section of the Community Medicine Department of Mt. Sinai Hospital in New York City, says that "Americans are on a collision course with hyperlipemia." The prefix *"hyper"* is from the Greek *"huper,"* meaning, literally, "too much." In colloquial terms, "hyperlipemia" is simply "too much fat in the blood plasma." Doctors are used to using these scientific blockbuster words, but I'm going to refer simply to "excess-fat-in-the-plasma."

In various parts of the United States, patient surveys are now being conducted to detect lipid abnormalities. Dr. Christakis found many hyperlipid people in the community, as did Dr. Kwiterovich of Johns Hopkins, who is also prominent in this field. However, the large medical centers are not the only ones involved in these surveys; people in the smaller places are also getting into it. Dr. Marvin L. Bierenbaum, director of the Atherosclerosis Research Group of St. Vincent's Hospital in Montclair, New Jersey, reports that his group is screening 1,000 to 1,500 persons annually. They find that about 40 percent of the patients they examine have some abnormality. In Rockland County, New York, Dr. Boris Vanadzin, County Commissioner of Health, started a countywide screening program and detected lipid abnormalities in 36 percent of the 1,635 men and women tested. The reports broke down as follows: 19.3 percent had excessive triglyceride levels; 6.5 percent showed high cholesterols; 10.2 percent had both abnormal triglyceride and cholesterol levels.

After lipid abnormalities have been detected by means of screenings such as I've described, the patients are referred to their own physicians, who will recommend the proper diet and medication for the specific type. Often diet is enough. In cases in which diet does not keep the condition under control, there are medications that are very helpful. But identifying and controlling the condition in adults is only one of the ways in which our newly gained knowledge of lipid abnormalities is being put to use.

Doctors have long been aware that heart disease tends to run in families. In 1897, Dr. William Osler, lecturing on angina pectoris, cited the Arnold family: William was a collector of customs; he died of "spasm of the heart." His son, Thomas, died of a heart attack. Thomas's famous son, Matthew, suffered for several years from heart disease before dying of a heart attack. Close relatives usually share a common environment, so it's not always safe to assume immediately that heredity is involved. However, by means of the typing tests we can now clearly demonstrate a genetic factor in atherosclerosis.

Dr. Joseph Goldstein did a very thorough study in Seattle, screening the plasma of 1,166 patients in thirteen hospitals over a period of eleven months. This figure represents 95 percent of all the patients who suffered acute myocardial infarctions in Seattle. They then followed 500 of the 885 patients who were still alive at the end of three months. They found that these 500 patients had a higher-than-average incidence of diabetes, obesity, and hypertension, and 31 percent had increased fats in their blood. In those under the age of forty this was so in a whopping 60 percent. Triglycerides were found to be elevated three times more often than cholesterol.

In the second phase of the Seattle study, 2,520 family members were tested. All were first-degree relatives: parents, brothers, sisters, and children. In this large group the average cholesterol level was 235, compared to a level in the control group of 218 (those with no family history of heart disease). Triglyceride level was 126, compared to the control level of 93. The investigators concluded that familial factors were clearly implicated. They then went on to study the death certificates of relatives who had died before the study was begun, and found twice as much coronary heart disease among families with hyperlipemia as among those without it.

Other studies have been undertaken by Dr. Goldstein, as a result of which he concludes that most people in the general population who have elevated cholesterol or triglyceride levels can't blame their troubles on heredity alone. He stresses what we've already discussed a number of times—the multifactorial basis of atherosclerosis. He feels that there is a large number of causes on which to blame most cases. It's highly possible, he hypothesizes, that the occurrence of premature coronary artery disease in these cases can be blamed on noxious environmental influences interacting with a gene that predisposes some people to excess-fat-in-the-plasma. It's not that more people are being born with these genes, but, as the environment (this includes diet, smoking, etc.) gets worse, the genes get more opportunity to exert their disastrous influence.

But there is a disease called "familial hyperlipemia" which is very definitely inherited. It occurs when the child gets the genetic trait from both sides of the family. Such children usually get heart disease at a young age and die before they have a chance to reproduce. Luckily most of us get high risk genetic material from only one parent.

Experiments with animals to determine the genetic patterns have been performed by Drs. T. B. Clarkson and H. B.

Lofland, Jr. They worked with a group of squirrel monkeys, giving them high-cholesterol feedings. On this diet, some of the monkeys loaded up their arteries with cholesterol. Some took on almost none. In between was a group of monkeys that stored only a little fat in their blood vessels. The investigators then did breeding experiments with the monkeys they'd raised. They mated pairs of monkeys from the group that had handled cholesterol most efficiently. Matings were also made between monkeys that had coped least well with the high-cholesterol diet. All the offspring received diets calculated to encourage development of atherosclerosis. In the next generation, all the animals with two parents that had been relatively unaffected by the diet took after their parents—they too were relatively unaffected. The children of the monkeys who filled their arteries with atherosclerotic plaques also developed atherosclerosis. Heredity was pretty well proved to be a factor.

Physicians have always been interested in prevention. However—and this is a very important however—up until now most of our effort has been toward what we call *secondary prevention*. This means trying to keep the disease from getting worse after it's been discovered. What we ought to be doing is bending our efforts toward *primary prevention* —finding people with predisposing factors as early in life as possible, and arranging matters so that disease never gets started.

The problem of identifying young children who have a high risk of early atherosclerosis was first tackled by Dr. Henry C. McGill of the University of Texas. He began with the microscopic examination of the arteries of young people who had been killed in accidents. He found streaks of fat on the surface of the aortas of teenagers. By late adolescence, he found, more substantial fat deposits had developed. In high-risk individuals in their twenties this fat was beginning to be incorporated into the substance of the arteries. By their thirties, this fat had hardened into well-developed fibrous plaques. A few more years and these plaques began to show calcification.

The question was whether early fat-streaking represents an early stage in the development of atherosclerosis. Many pathologists are cooperating in an International Atherosclerosis Project. Some 23,000 sets of coronary arteries were studied, all over the world. The pathologists found streaks of fat in the coronary arteries of children and adolescents of some fourteen countries. However, fibrous plaques and complicated lesions occurred frequently only in populations where there is a great deal of early death from coronary disease. The doctors agreed that the early fatty streaks found in children may do one of three things: they may regress, stay the same, or develop to form plaques. Which of these three possibilities takes place depends mostly on how much lipid is in the streaks. The amount of lipid depends on dietary patterns and heredity. Among American combat casualties in Vietnam—soldiers with a mean age of twenty-two— some atherosclerosis was found in 45 percent and severe coronary disease in 5 percent!

Right now we're beginning to study the problem even earlier. You may be surprised when I tell you that it is possible to run the test for Type II disorders on blood from the umbilical cord at birth, and that's precisely what's being done in newborns with a family history of early heart disease. By the time a baby is twenty-four hours old, its pediatrician has the results. We hope these tests on newborns will eventually be routine. By law it is necessary to test now for a disease known as phenylketonuria, yet this is thousands of times less common than atherosclerosis. Once a pediatrician is aware of the situation, the infant can be started immediately on the proper formula.

Several screening projects are currently being sponsored by the National Heart and Lung Institute to determine whether risk factors associated with coronary heart disease in adults can be detected early. School children being tested in Muscatine, Iowa, and in Rochester, Minnesota, are from families in which one parent has had a myocardial infarction by the age of fifty. So far there are 94 families with 243 children in the study; it is anticipated that, ultimately, 500 children will be studied for at least five years. Each child is examined three times during the first month, and then at less frequent but regular intervals. Some children show normal blood-lipid levels; others are already abnormal. In seven of the first forty-five, the cholesterol level was above 250; in two of them, above 350. Most of these children come from families with Type II problems.

It's too soon, of course, to be at all sure that putting high-risk infants on diets will ensure their growing up with normal arteries. So far all we have is the ability to identify them, but it's a good start. This new "pediatric approach" is being used by Dr. Charles J. Glueck and his group at Cincinnati General Hospital. They've screened 3,800 newborns so far, obtaining blood by the umbilical method. They found twenty infants with Type II. All of them had one parent with the same Type II. An affiliated private hospital turned up another fourteen infants. All thirty-four of these babies were placed on low-cholesterol, high-polyunsaturate diets. The children did well until they were about six years old. As they grew older, drug therapy had to be added to keep down cholesterol levels.

Dr. Glueck reported that the parents' problem was often not diagnosed until after its discovery in the newborn. In the family of one such newborn, the thirty-five-year-old mother was found to have a Type II disorder. Of her three other children, an eight-year-old showed Type II excess blood fat, and a two-year-old's tests were borderline. The maternal grandmother had died at the age of thirty-six of acute myocardial infarction.

An extreme case has been reported from Mercy Catholic Medical Center in Philadelphia. A seven-year-old boy with a 769 cholesterol, who was not overweight, had already had anginal chest pains. His father had died of a heart attack at thirty-two. Two uncles had died of heart attacks, one at thirty-six, the other at fifty-two; an aunt who had died at fifty had a cholesterol of 910. Five of this boy's seven brothers and sisters had elevated cholesterol levels. The Philadelphia doctors put all these youngsters on low-cholesterol diets. The higher the cholesterol at the outset, the greater was the effect of the diet. The seven-year-old's cholesterol was cut by 49 percent. However, it was still much too high, so drugs were prescribed. His level has since dropped 58 percent, but it's still elevated. Maybe now, with the new techniques, he could have been treated from birth.

One of the most extensive family programs I know of is the one in Arizona, where 10,000 families with preschool children have already been enlisted. Dr. Glenn M. Friedman of Scottsdale (Arizona) and his colleagues are trying to teach these families the importance of proper diet and exercise. Dr. Friedman's initial tests of the first 1,771 families showed that 16 percent of the children—or a little better than one in every six—already had a cholesterol level of 160. "If this trend continues," Dr. Friedman said, "this disease will be the cause of death of 50 percent of our children, and for countless thousands it will be in young life." On the diet program, of the 276 children with high cholesterol who were retested after a few months, 68 percent showed a decrease of at least 10 percent in cholesterol levels.

There's no need to go into more detail of programs being advocated by doctors in various parts of the country who are at work on the problem of atherosclerosis in children, for all of them encompass the same recommendations I've been making in this book. There's only one further piece of advice I want to offer here: Don't wait for your doctor to test your children. Ask him to do it. It's of vital importance to their future.

6

Eating Habits—Practical Ways to Change for the Better

"WE ARE A NATION of nutritional illiterates. Despite a wealth of scientific knowledge of nutrition, too many of us do not know what a balanced diet is, and we are ignorant of the essential nutrients we need and the foods that contain them. We have an abundant food supply, yet our eating habits are deteriorating. And it is not just the poor who are affected. The U.S. Department of Agriculture reports that the percentage of households that met or exceeded the department's definition of a good diet dropped from 60 to 50 percent from 1955 to 1965. Nine percent of families with incomes over $10,000 had diets rated poor."

These are not my words, but the words of Henry J. Heinz II, chairman of the H. J. Heinz Company. He's saying, of course, that the proper foods are available, but too many people don't want them. He is not saying, though he well might, that the food manufacturing industry, by its constant advertising and production of junk foods, has not distinguished itself by contributing much to nutritional literacy, or even good nutritional habits.

Poor nutrition can start before birth, while the infant is still in the uterus. If the mother is eating improperly, the development of the fetus will be adversely affected. Unfortunately, many mothers who are careful to eat the right foods during

44

pregnancy don't feed their babies properly. Poor nutrition often starts immediately after birth. Too many babies start out with a nutritional handicap: they aren't fed human milk, and that's what they should be getting—not cow's milk. Cow's milk is different in many important respects from human milk. Cow's milk contains 3.5 grams of protein in every 100 milliliters; human milk contains only 1.1 grams of protein. In other words, there's just about three times as much protein in cow's milk. A calf doubles its birthweight in 50 days, while an infant needs 150 days to double its birthweight. The calf gains three times as fast, which correlates perfectly with the triple amount of protein it gets from its mother's milk. There are many different kinds of protein. Cow's milk has the proper balance of proteins for cows. Human milk has the proper balance for humans.

As for fats, human milk contains a predominance of monounsaturated fatty acids. On the other hand, cow's milk contains mostly saturated fatty acids. That's why some babies are intolerant of these fats and don't absorb them well.

In other words, what the infant is fed will affect its health as an adult. Doctors have always known that babies do best on mothers' milk. If that's not feasible, they should be given one of the new prepared formulas that conform as closely as possible to the composition of human milk. The old-fashioned formulas, which consisted of cow's milk diluted with water and with added table sugar, or corn syrup, are inadequate.

In Chapter 7 I will explain at some length how crucial it is to prevent overweight from getting a start in babies, at the time the fat cells are being formed. Breast-feeding is an important factor in the prevention of obesity in the infant. Dr. Lewis A. Barness of the University of Pennsylvania points out that bottle-fed babies are more likely to be subjected to a subtle form of pressure to finish what's in the bottle, whereas breast-fed babies are usually allowed to stop eating when they stop sucking.

Each pediatrician has his own answer to the question of how long women should continue to breast-feed. Many believe that at least six months is essential, because the infant's ability to absorb human milk fat and most vegetable oils is good, while his ability to absorb butterfat is limited. Some doctors prefer mothers to continue to breast-feed their babies through the first nine months of life.

When the baby is switched from mother's milk to cow's milk, should the switch be to whole or to skim milk? This is a question that is being hotly debated by researchers who hold conflicting views. Some are convinced that skim milk is perfectly all right for a four-month-old baby, while others say skim milk is bad for children under two. I'll give you both points of view.

Dr. Samuel J. Foman, professor of pediatrics at the University of Iowa Medical College, thinks that children under two should not drink skim milk. He says his research shows that on a diet of skim milk a baby's calorie intake is inadequate, his protein intake is excessive, his fat intake is much too low, and so is his intake of certain necessary fatty acids. Dr. Foman advises changing over from whole milk to skim milk when the child reaches the age of two.

So much for Dr. Foman and the case in favor of whole milk for children under two. We now come to the diametrically opposed views of Dr. Glenn Friedman of Scottsdale, Arizona, and his colleague, Dr. Stanley J. Goldberg, professor of pediatrics at the University of Arizona. These two doctors studied two groups of children—fifty-two patients of Dr. Friedman's and fifty-two similar patients from the practice of another pediatrician—as a control group. Dr. Friedman switched all his patients to skim milk at the age of four months, when he put them all on a low-cholesterol, low-saturated-fat diet. It was found that all the children in the study had significantly lower cholesterol levels than those in the control group, and that their growth and development were not adversely affected. All the youngsters in the study were evaluated every six months for a number of factors, including height, weight, head circumference, skinfold thickness, motor and language development, and so on.

How can two groups of pediatricians achieve such widely differing results? One explanation might be that Dr. Friedman's children received other foods in addition to their skim milk, and so got the nutritional elements they needed from solid foods.

I tend to prefer a position somewhere in between the two extremes represented by Drs. Foman and Friedman. It's probably a good idea to switch normal babies from whole to skim milk when they're about a year old, but the precise time to make the switch should depend upon the individual baby. It's best to follow the advice of your own doctor in making this decision. After all, he or she knows your baby; many factors must be considered before making a recommendation, including the family's history of heart disease and the child's cholesterol level. I'm talking here about typical, healthy children only.

Most doctors agree that children from the age of two on do best on skim milk. If whole milk is continued, no more than a pint a day should be used. That old adage about a quart of milk every day has been found to be—like so many old wives' tales —a lot of nonsense.

Many of my readers may argue this point because they have been brought up to believe that the richer the milk, the better. There's a good reason why your parents received this erroneous impression. Before the days of government regulation of dairy products, many farmers adulterated their milk with water, without telling the consumer. As a consequence many children suffered from malnutrition. Because of this common abuse, a regulation was placed on the books stating that milk must have a butterfat content of at least 4 percent. While I agree that the government is right in insisting that milk be correctly labeled, I know that all this butterfat is not good for children past the age of two.

Another old wives' tale that should be discredited is the idea that a fat baby is a healthy baby. It simply isn't so. A generation ago diaper services rented infant scales to customers. Mothers weighed their babies once a week and bragged to each other about weight gains. The baby who'd logged the highest number of ounces was regarded with envy and admiration by the mothers of all the other infants. About the time the disposable diaper came in, the home baby scale went out. It's as old-fashioned as the flannel petticoat.

Perhaps you feel I'm belaboring the point. Well, so I am. I do it because I feel it is impossible to overemphasize the importance of letting the *baby* decide how much it wili eat. Offer it a balanced diet of the foods that are good for it, and when it indicates that it's had enough, remove the bottle or plate. There's nothing intrinsically good about a "clean" plate. We used to hear a lot about "the starving Armenians." Parents tried to make their children feel guilty if every bite wasn't consumed. As if there were any way of conveying the uneaten food to hungry children in Armenia—or anywhere else! Today's up-to-date, aware parents know that teaching children to overeat is the road to a lifetime of overweight, with a strong likelihood that the child will develop atherosclerosis.

Sometimes healthy children will go along for several days "eating like birds." Then, for a few meals, they'll eat a great deal. Over a period of time it will balance out. So long as your child is offered only foods that are good for him or her, the best way is to let the child be the judge of how much—or how little —it wants to eat.

Dr. Glenn Friedman stresses the importance of discouraging children from nibbling and snacking between meals. Children can only adjust themselves when they are offered balanced meals at regular intervals. If a child is allowed to help itself to a bag of potato chips at two o'clock, a candy bar at three, and a package of cookies at four, that child won't want to eat a well-balanced dinner at six.

The time to teach a child to eat healthful foods at regular intervals is while it is still too young to have any say in these matters. Then, when it's older, it is more likely to do what it's been used to doing.

If when you were growing up your parents thought it made meat more palatable to cover it with extra salt and ketchup, you probably learned to do the same thing. Even if you now serve undoctored meat to your children, they'll watch you jazzing up your own portion, and they'll get the impression that that's a desirable thing to do—something they too can do when they're grown up. But when they see you eating properly, they'll take it for granted that that's the right way to eat.

So much for habit training. Now let's move on to what specific foods are going to be served at your table. I'm not talking now about a diet. "Diets" are for people who are sick. I'm talking about lifetime patterns of eating.

Most people eat too much. The average American adult eats more than 3,000 calories a day. We ought to get our caloric intake down where it belongs—to 2,400 calories daily or possibly even lower, depending upon the individual metabolism. The Inter-Society Commission for Heart Disease Resources recently recommended that people eat less than 300 milligrams of cholesterol each day, that the total calories of fat be kept to less than 35 percent of the diet, and that these fats be divided equally among saturated, monounsaturated, and polyunsaturated sources.

This advice isn't of much use to the family cook. Translated into action, what does it mean? The American Heart Association recommends a daily consumption of:

- Two cups of low-fat milk or low-fat milk products—low-fat cheese, low-fat ice cream, etc.
- Six ounces of fish, poultry, or lean meat, or its equivalent in a vegetable protein such as beans.
- At least two cups of vegetables and fruits (including a mixture of dark green and bright yellow vegetables).
- At least four servings of breads or cereals of the whole grain or enriched variety.
- Two to four tablespoonsful of polyunsaturated fats or oils.

How can you tell which fats are polyunsaturated? As I mentioned earlier, most of the liquid vegetable oils are polyunsaturated, including soybean, corn, cottonseed, sesame seed, and safflower oil. These oils tend to lower the cholesterol level. Olive oil and peanut oil are both liquid and of vegetable origin, but they're *mono*unsaturated. In other words, they may not plug up the arteries as rapidly as saturated fats do, but neither do they lower cholesterol. As for coconut oil, it's as high in saturated fat as butter. When the label on a package tells you the product contains "vegetable oil," it doesn't necessarily follow that all of the oil in the product is one of the polyunsaturated or monounsaturated fats. Some of that vegetable oil may be saturated.

The fats to avoid are animal fats: butterfat, meat fats, and particularly such animal fats as lard, bacon fat, and other pork products.

It's simple enough to cut the fat off the edges of a piece of steak or a slice of ham. You cannot cut the fat off bologna, salami, hot dogs, piecrust, Danish pastry—or any other product that has fat mixed all through it. The Commission for Heart Disease Resources urged the food industry to make available leaner processed meats, and dairy products, frozen desserts, and baked goods that are lower in saturated fats and cholesterol. Pressure from consumers is going to be necessary if this project is to succeed. The commission has recommended that policies and regulations be reviewed and revised to achieve a number of objectives. They are:

- Development of animals whose meat has a lower fat content than we find in the supermarket today. As you probably know, cattle are kept in pens and fattened before they're slaughtered. Meat would be cheaper as well as healthier for your family if this practice were stopped. While you can trim the fat off the edges of your steak, you can't cut out the marbling of fat that you'll find clear through it.
- Modernization of rules and regulations having to do with

meat products. There are actually laws that processed meats can't be made with vegetable oils. The Food and Drug Administration and the Department of Agriculture define the use of vegetable oils as "adulteration." These rules were made before doctors knew what they've recently learned about the evils of saturated fats. It's going to take time and effort by the public to get these laws changed.

- Reduction of the saturated fats used in commercial baked goods. If the consumer learns to ask for bakery items made with unsaturated fat and to reject those that don't fit his requirements, the industry will soon switch.
- Reduction of the saturated fats in cheese, ice cream, and cream substitutes. More and more skim-milk cheeses are coming on the market. It is now possible to buy ice milk or sherbet in preference to ice cream. But learn how to read labels before you purchase any of these products. For example, some cream substitutes are made from coconut oil, which is one of the most potent agents for raising the amount of cholesterol in the blood. A label reading "made with vegetable oil" implies that the product is better for you than one made with dairy fat, but that's not necessarily true. You need to go one step further and find out what kind of vegetable oil has been used. Coconut oil and hydrogenated (hardened) vegetable oils are just as bad for your arteries as cream.

Here's a summary of the recommendations of the Inter-Society Commission for Heart Disease for changing your family's eating habits to achieve better nutrition:

- Use lean cuts of meat (beef, lamb, pork, veal) cooked in such a way that the saturated fats they contain are cooked out. Serve no more than five moderate-sized portions weekly.
- Use only processed meat products (hot dogs, cold cuts, etc.) made with reduced amounts of saturated fats.
- Use very few organ meats (liver, kidney, etc.) and shellfish.
- Avoid bacon (except lean Canadian bacon), lard, suet, and

egg yolk (no more than three whole eggs a week for adults, seven for children).

• Use more lean poultry and fish.
• Use low-fat and fat-modified dairy products.
• Use fat-modified baked goods and candies.
• Use salad oils, cooking oils, and soft margarines instead of butter and shortenings high in saturated fat.
• Use grains, fruits, vegetables, and legumes (beans and peas).

FOODS HIGH IN CHOLESTEROL ARE: Egg yolk, organ meats (liver, kidney), dairy products (butter, cream, cheeses made with whole milk, ice cream), shellfish (clams, oysters).

FOODS LOW IN CHOLESTEROL ARE: Skim milk, cheeses made with skim milk, egg white, soft margarine, vegetable oils that are low in saturated fats, peanut butter, legumes (beans and peas), vegetables, fruits, whole-grain cereals and breads.

A convenient summary of this information is published in a folder entitled "The Way To A Man's Heart." For a copy of this excellent little publication, write to the American Heart Association, 44 East 23rd Street, New York, N.Y. 10010.

Teaching your children to eat sensibly is not simply a matter of serving well-balanced, nutritious meals and letting the kids see you practicing what you preach in the way of eating habits. You will have to fight constant pressure from outside your home. In fact, these pressures often enter your home—in the shape of TV commercials that urge your children to "ask Mommy to buy chocolate snerdles for your breakfast."

How do you prevent your children from joining the ranks of the snackers who fill up with potato chips and sugary snacks? First of all, don't buy these products; then there won't be any on your shelves. What do you do when Johnny complains, in the late afternoon, that he's "starving"? Offer him carrot sticks, apple slices, a stalk of celery, or a handful of raisins or raw string beans. Very small children consider such foods a treat. Once they've developed a taste for crunchy raw fruits and vegetables, it will stick with them for the rest of their lives.

When children grow older, it's much harder to keep them eating correctly. When they go with the gang to a hamburger stand, there's no way to prevent them from ordering the cheeseburgers and French fries the other kids are having. But you can make sure your teenagers understand the importance of proper nutrition and hope they'll eat the wrong foods only occasionally, when they're out with their peers.

It's estimated that the average teenager eats one-fourth of his or her daily food in snacks. I hope you'll do all you can in the way of education (not nagging) to ensure that your child won't grow into one of those adults whose idea of a healthful meal is two martinis, a fat-marbled steak, a baked potato with sour cream, and a tossed salad with Roquefort dressing—followed by an evening of TV watching, accompanied by beer and pretzels.

One of the strangest paradoxes in our affluent society is the way we feed our dogs as compared to the diet we offer our children—not to mention ourselves. The owner of a pedigreed dog is very careful to offer him a well-balanced diet. That dog owner makes sure his dog has a shiny coat, doesn't grow too fat, gets enough regular exercise. Meanwhile, the dog owners' kids are sitting in front of the TV set, munching empty-calorie snacks. The dog isn't allowed to eat that junk!

Many people are now beginning to see the absurdity of this behavior. As is usual with reformers, the advocates of healthful natural foods have gone a bit far in their insistence on organically grown natural foods. They've turned off a great many potential converts with their talk of soybean croquettes and carrot-juice cocktails. When a pendulum starts to swing in the opposite direction, it almost always swings too far. This is a shame, because the reformers are right when they shout that we are eating incorrectly. I hope you aren't going to ignore everything I've been telling you simply because you've been turned off by a friend who is a "diet nut." Your friend may well go too far, but the basic point is well taken. Nature presents food to us in a perfect package. Once we start monkeying with it, we deplete its "trophic" value.

What's trophic value? That's a food's ability to promote its own correct usage as fuel for the body's cells and tissues. According to Roger J. Williams of the University of Texas, foods must furnish both the calories and the raw materials needed to build and maintain the body's metabolic machinery. Williams says that it is easy enough to measure calories, but what he calls the "beyond-calorie" quality of food—its trophic value—is difficult to measure. (Trophic value is measured by feeding laboratory animals the substance to be tested and noting the rate at which the animal grows and develops sexually. Animals develop more slowly when fed foods with low trophic values.) Nutrients function as a team or a chain in which no links can be missing, Williams says. As an example, he gives "enriched" white bread, which shows up well in tables that list food composition because it's been enriched with the items that are usually emphasized in such lists. However, the bread's trophic value may actually be much lower. Other items not included in the tables are either not contained in the bread or are not present in the correct quantities. Bread made from natural flour has a much higher trophic value than does packaged bread, he found.

Trophic value is not the only aspect of processed grain being questioned by nutritionists. The fiber content of whole grains is also being studied. A British investigator, Dr. Denis Burkitt, is convinced that when fiber consumption is high, the cholesterol level falls; conversely, the cholesterol level rises as the amount of fiber in the diet is reduced. Dr. Burkitt, who was a surgeon in Uganda for some twenty years, found that Africans, on their native diet, eliminated the residue of a meal in about thirty-five hours. Englishmen take seventy-seven to one hundred hours to eliminate residue. Undoubtedly you've heard many times that the roughage in cereals is an aid to elimination, but the extension of this concept—connecting fiber, or roughage, with cholesterol levels—is something new. Dr. Burkitt has a theory, linking the swifter passage through the intestinal tract of the residue from natural grains to the metabolism of bile acids. He believes that when more bile acids are excreted, cholesterol levels are lower.

It's too soon to do more than outline these theories, since few studies have been done on them and there is basic disagreement among members of the medical profession. For instance, Dr. Ernst L. Wynder, president of the American Health Foundation, thinks it's the low-fat content of the Africans' diet that is responsible for their lower cholesterol levels. Time—and further research—will tell.

You probably feel I've been pretty cavalier in my sweeping recommendations that you change your lifetime habits. It's not too difficult to alter your children's eating patterns, but readjusting your own is tough. After all, you learned them when you yourself were very young and you've had them for years. It's all very well for me to demand, "Cut down on the amount of red meat you eat," but it's no fun at all for you to pass up the steak on the restaurant menu in favor of fish. So I'm happy to be able to end this section on a comparatively optimistic note by telling you that, so far as beef, lamb, and milk products are concerned, there's a good chance that these products may one day be less harmful, without any effort on the part of the consumer. In several countries scientists are working to "polyunsaturate the ruminant animals on the hoof," as a reporter for *Medical World News* has written.

In Ireland, Dr. J. F. Connolly of the Agricultural Institute in Castleknock has been testing a new feeding technique he thinks has significantly raised the polyunsaturated fat level of the meat of experimental lambs. In Australia, Dr. Paul J. Nestel of the National University in Canberra is using a different technique on cows, in the hope of achieving milk with a high level of polyunsaturates. A team of scientists in Wooster, Ohio, is working on still another way of altering cow's milk. So, you see, the future looks brighter.

As I pointed out at the beginning of this chapter, the ideal diet would be the one followed by our cavemen ancestors: fruits, vegetables, cereals, and nuts; lean meat, fish, and fowl, cooked either by roasting or baking—all without the addition of salt. (I'll be talking about the evils of too much salt in Chapter 10.) I wish I could believe that I've convinced you to return to such a safe, sensible way of eating. However, through the years I've watched my patients reverting to their old bad habits as their fear of heart attack and imminent death began to fade.

It's small wonder that people backslide if they get no cooperation from the cook, who doesn't understand the need to change a lifetime's cooking habits. You can't expect a patient to enjoy a meal of low-cholesterol fish, vegetables, and a dessert orange while the rest of the family is eating steak, French fries, green beans cooked with bacon, and coconut-custard pie. Unless that man or woman is either afraid for his/her life or more than normally strong-willed, there's bound to be a rebellion.

I am therefore going to address myself to the family menu planner and cook. In some families that person is still a full-time housewife, while in others husband and wife now share K.P. duties, with older boys and girls getting into the act. No matter who's in charge—husband, wife, or family committee—you should start thinking in terms of improving the health and lengthening the lives of everybody in your family. Even if you can't quite see yourselves as cave dwellers, there are still many less-radical ways to improve your eating habits.

I think it's safe to assume that you wouldn't be reading this book if you weren't concerned about the risk of heart attack. Your concern should take the form of a rethinking of your basic attitudes toward what goes on in your kitchen.

Instead of putting one person on a strict, boring diet and continuing to cook for the rest of the family just the way you've always done, I hope you'll set about changing your basic philosophy. That sounds very radical, but once you've readjusted your thinking, you're not going to find it nearly as traumatic as you expected. And you'll find it pays rich dividends. Your new culinary philosophy is not only better for the adults, it's also better for your children, who should become accustomed to proper eating habits—unless you want to see them develop atherosclerotic plaques, too. Of course, you don't want anything of the kind.

I'm going to turn the last couple of pages of this chapter over to my collaborator, who tells me she's learned a lot about cooking for a family on a low-cholesterol diet since her own husband had a heart attack. I'll leave you cooking experts to have a talk.

* * *

The revolution has to start in the supermarket. Leave the cream, butter, homogenized milk, and lard on the shelves. That's right. No butter is to be served at your table, not even to guests. You may be in for a surprise. As you pass your visitors the tub of soft margarine, you're likely to hear, "So you've given up butter, have you? We use margarine at home, too."

Don't sneer at margarine. You're probably thinking of the old hardened margarines, which had an unpleasant consistency and a worse flavor. Times have changed. The new soft margarines are quite palatable. Try different brands until you find one that you and your family like.

Soft margarine is a table spread. Its flavor alters when it's heated in a frying pan. It is not a good substitute for butter when it comes to cooking. Instead, use one of the polyunsaturated vegetable oils.

As you know, it's impossible to remove any of the fat from homogenized milk. Instant nonfat dry milk is not only much cheaper than homogenized milk, it also has the advantage of keeping indefinitely in the package, and it tastes fine—if properly used. If you drink it immediately after it's been mixed with water, dry milk tastes exactly like powdered chalk! It needs to stand for several hours, and preferably overnight, in the refrigerator. Few children object to drinking skim milk. For adults who can't get used to it, turn to one of the commercial skim milks to which a very small quantity of whole milk has been added. Or you can do it yourself by adding a little whole milk to the powdered milk after you've mixed it.

As for eggs, you already know it's the yolk that's cholesterol-laden. The white of the egg is guiltless. So far, the egg substitutes on the market—advertisements to the contrary notwithstanding—do not taste very much like whole egg. However, they work very well in cooked foods that don't depend primarily upon the flavor of egg yolk. If you use them for making scrambled eggs, you'll have to add something with a strong flavor of its own to disguise the taste—chives, for instance.

You'll be pleased to find how many of your favorite recipes you can continue to use if you make just a few adjustments in them. And you may also be surprised at how little difference most of these changes will make in the results. Here are some of the ways in which you can cut down on the cholesterol content of your meals without doing violence to your reputation as a good cook:

- Spaghetti sauce — After you've cooked the hamburger until all the red color is gone, pour the contents of the frying pan into a colander and drain off all the fat. Now continue with your regular recipe.
- Soups, stews, and casseroles — Prepare these dishes a day ahead of time. Refrigerate overnight. Skim off the fat that rises to the top. If you like to thicken them with flour or cornstarch, wait to do that until you've removed the fat.
- Sautéed foods — Invest in a teflon frying pan, in which you can sauté with much less oil. Instead of the butter you used to use, substitute cooking oil. In those rare cases where the flavor of butter is indispensable (for mushrooms, for instance) add a teaspoonful of butter to the salad oil. That way you get the flavor without most of the cholesterol.
- Cheese — There are a number of cheeses made with skim milk, including mozzarella and a Norwegian cheese called Jarlsberg. Ask your local cheese store for help in finding new cheeses you can substitute in your old recipes. You don't have to stop serving lasagna, for instance; just substitute skim-milk mozzarella and leave out the ricotta. It won't be as rich, but it's still good. In parts of northern Italy, very little cheese is used in lasagna; instead, Italian cooks use a cream sauce—which you can make very successfully with skim milk.
- Chocolate — Although rich chocolate is taboo on low-cholesterol diets, cocoa is okay and can be substituted in many recipes. Three tablespoons of cocoa is the equivalent of an ounce of baking chocolate.
- Bacon and salt-pork — Many cooks depend heavily on pork products for flavoring vegetables. If you are one of them, try adding imitation bacon bits after the vegetable is cooked. These bacon bits are also good in salads. Here again, some brands are much better than others, so please don't give up if you don't like the first one you try.

A little wine is a fine low-cholesterol way to add flavor to stews, casseroles, and sauces. If you're not used to cooking with wine, here's a bit of advice: Always simmer the sauce long enough to get rid of the alcoholic taste.

Herbs can make otherwise boring foods into delicious dishes. Every supermarket has a wide variety of dried herbs in jars. Undoubtedly you are already familiar with some of them. Now's the time to explore the more exotic ones. There are a number of herb cookbooks on the market. There are also low-cholesterol cookbooks. Several of these are available in inexpensive paperback editions, but most local libraries have cookbooks which you can consult for free. Many of the recipes won't appeal to you, but you can probably find a few in each book to substitute for the old favorites. And as you pursue your researches you're almost certain to discover some new ones.

7

Obesity–
Eating Your Way to Sickness

A FEW DAYS AGO one of my patients told me he'd looked into a straight life insurance policy for $25,000. His insurance agent had told him that the average premium was $575 for a man his age (thirty-five) with normal weight and blood pressure. Unfortunately for my patient, he's 50 pounds overweight, which is going to add $72.25 to his premium. His systolic pressure, instead of being 130, is 160, and that's going to add another $108.25. The extra charges were bad enough, but what really upset this man was hearing that instead of the normal longevity of thirty-nine years predicted by the agent's tables, his longevity was ten years less because of the complications I've mentioned. He said he could understand why the insurance company was concerned about the elevated blood pressure, but the obesity didn't make sense to him. He told me indignantly that a couple of his father's friends were fat—and in the best of health.

To a certain extent, he's right. Obesity by itself doesn't seem to be a risk factor in heart attack and sudden death. But many fat people have atherosclerosis, hypertension, diabetes, gallbladder disease, and other maladies. Obesity rarely occurs alone; it aggravates the other factors, and avoiding it is important.

Now let me be clear about what I mean when I say obesity.

Lots of people think the word *obese* means "really fat." Not so. A healthy man shouldn't be even a little fat—not even enough to joke about that tire around his middle. If he is, there's no sense calling him "a little on the heavy side." He's obese. And obesity is a sign of poor health.

Our ideas about obesity have changed a great deal in recent years. There was a time when your doctor weighed and measured you, then found the ideal weight for an individual of your age, sex, height, and weight by locating the correct figure on a chart. These charts had been compiled by insurance companies, using averages arrived at by weighing and measuring large numbers of people.

Now we know that such "correct" figures are often incorrect. Take Joe Namath. He's six-feet-two and his playing weight is 200 pounds. According to those old insurance-company charts, Joe Namath is at least 20 pounds overweight. But I defy you to find a spare ounce of fat on his muscular athlete's body. You see, the difficulty is that muscle weighs more than fat. Some charts take no account of this fact, nor of the fact that Joe has broad shoulders and big bones.

Unfortunately, some people think you ought to document everything. That's nonsense. You don't have to be a doctor to diagnose whether somebody is fat. Most of the time you can tell just by taking a good look. Today's criterion for the designation of obesity is the amount of subcutaneous fat tissue (fat tissue under the skin), not the weight. The fat under the skin can be estimated well enough by an experienced doctor. He simply pinches the proper places. These diagnostic spots are the triceps (the back of the upper arm, halfway between shoulder and elbow) and the back, just below the shoulder blades. If he wants to judge obesity more accurately, instead of pinching with his fingers he can pinch with a calipers—large forceps marked off in millimeters.

If you want to get really fancy about it you can go to the densitometric method. This is based on the low specific gravity of adipose tissue (fat). Archimedes first stated the principle involved—that of weighing people first in air and then in water. You can get involved in a lot of complicated figures if you want to, but it usually isn't necessary.

When my patients ask me how much weight they ought to lose, I say, "Keep losing until you can't pick up a fold of your belly anymore." Here's a very practical test for a man: If your waist measurement is greater than your chest measurement, you are significantly overweight. Unfortunately, this test won't work for a woman, but it's not significant. (Any woman can tell at a glance if another female is too fat. You don't have to be a doctor.) For anyone whose weight was ideal at age twenty to twenty-five and who was in good physical condition at that time, that same weight would be ideal at age forty, fifty, or sixty.

Dr. Jean Mayer of Harvard, the well-known nutrition specialist, points out that in animal husbandry, when a fat animal was desired, the following procedures were used: For hogs and cattle, an obese strain was selected. For oxen and capons, castration was employed. Chickens were injected with estrogens (female sex hormones), and estrogen pellets were implanted in cattle (until it became illegal). Animals were cooped up or penned up to prevent them from getting any exercise.

Obviously, farmers know that heredity, hormones, and lack of exercise are all important factors in obesity.

There are many different reasons for overweight, not just one. We used to think it was all very simple: If you ate too much, you got too fat; thin people were people who knew when to stop eating. We no longer believe that. Surely you know people who can eat whatever they like, stuffing themselves if they are so inclined, but who never gain an ounce. You also know some who claim they can gain weight just by looking at a slice of cake. Unless you yourself are one of them, you probably thought they were secret eaters. It's not so in most cases.

The cause of overweight may be due to one or to a combination of factors. These include:

- Heredity
- Abnormal metabolism
- Psychological factors
- An impairment of the mechanism in the brain, often referred to as the "appestat," that regulates food intake
- Physical inactivity

Heredity is certainly one of the more important factors. Although obesity occurs in all physical types, it occurs with greater frequency in some than in others. Doctors recognize three basic body types.

The ectomorph, at one end of the human scale, is fragile, thin, linear, with a small body and long arms and legs. Ectomorphs tend to be slender, with comparatively delicate bone structure and stringy muscular development. It's almost impossible for them to get fat.

At the other end of the scale are the endomorphs, with large bodies and short arms and legs. This type is most inclined to overweight. The abdomen is more massive than the shoulder-chest area. Endomorphs tend to be soft, round, obese.

In between these two extremes, we have the mesomorph, who is hard and square. This type has a massive, muscular chest and prominent body joints.

Most people are not pure types. Most of us are a combination of these three basic types, but have more characteristics of one than of the others. Most obese persons are inherently endomorphic. Dr. Mayer thinks endomorphy is an inherited predisposition to the laying on of fat unless insufficient diet, great activity, disease, or voluntary weight control supervenes. He made this statement in connection with obesity in young adolescents, adding that the obesity problem in adults is far more complex.

Middle-aged persons are inclined to blossom suddenly into obesity. One day Joe Namath will quit playing football. By the time he's in his fifties, he'll very likely be carrying as much as one-third more fat, without gaining much weight. You've probably noticed that most middle-aged former athletes have paunches. That's because some of the muscle has been replaced by fat. This process can go in the other direction, however. Many times I've had a patient who's been on an exercise program climb onto the scale, do a double take, and protest: "How come I haven't lost any weight? The scale says I weigh the same, but look at my pants. They're falling off, they're so big around the waist." He is right, of course. He's replaced some of his fat with muscle, which is heavier. That's why scale weight is not the answer.

Most doctors are fairly well agreed that heredity is one of the primary causes of obesity. Studies have shown that with normal-weight parents, only 7 percent of children are obese. If one parent is obese, then 40 percent of the children will be overweight. And if both parents are overweight, 80 percent of their children will be, too. Researchers wondered if poor eating habits don't have a lot to do with these statistics. They investigated and found that adopted children had no correlation at all with the weights of their foster parents. Environment, in this instance, was not as important as body build. But environment certainly is important. The habits of eating learned early in life tend to establish patterns that may be followed forever. In some societies, obesity is looked on with favor; the eating habits are responsible to a large extent for keeping the weight up to the socially acceptable level.

We don't need to spend much time on the factor known as "metabolic obesity," in which the primary lesion is an error—either inborn or acquired—in tissue metabolism. We're not talking about derangements in metabolism, but about the average person. Many obese persons would prefer to believe that their overweight is due to some factor such as a sluggish thyroid gland and dream of pounds melting away as they make no other effort than that of swallowing a few pills. Unfortunately, such situations are the exception rather than the rule. Patients who really do suffer from a metabolic dysfunction will be correctly diagnosed and treated by their doctors.

For a good many years now it has been fashionable to blame obesity on psychosomatic factors. Amateur psychiatrists are prone to remark, "No wonder she's fat. She's comforting herself with food because her father ignored her when she was a child." There are, of course, plenty of authentic cases in which patients overeat because they are depressed. However, at least as many moderately obese persons have completely normal personalities. Their psychological difficulties related to overweight arise only if pressure is put on them to reduce. Obese children also cause a good deal of strife within the family, but, oddly enough, corrective measures are almost never instituted until psychosocial problems appear. It's very important not to wait for older children to develop social problems, but to get started early. Children shouldn't be made to feel "different." That's where the psychiatric problems start. To think that the average moderately obese person is overweight because of psychiatric problems is putting the cart before the horse. It's the obesity that causes the problem, not the other way around.

Dr. Albert Stunkard of the University of Pennsylvania found a certain amount of relationship between emotional disturbance and obesity. He found a far more striking relationship between social class and obesity. Cheap foods are fattening, and people with lower incomes must use more of them to get calories. How much do you pay for a pound of meat or fish compared to a pound of spaghetti? One more finding by this same physician was that in the upper classes, whatever neuroses young obese women may have are inclined to be closely related to their obesity. That would seem to indicate that they developed neuroses because they were fat, not that they became fat as a result of neurosis.

Dr. Stunkard reported another interesting study of the differences in eating habits between obese and nonobese persons when availability of food was a factor. The subjects were not told that the tests involved their eating habits. Obese and nonobese subjects were tested separately, but under identical conditions. In one test, a plate containing one sandwich was placed before each test subject. He was told that if he wanted more, there were sandwiches in the refrigerator nearby. In the second test, three sandwiches were placed on the plate, with more available in the refrigerator.

Here's the way it worked out: In the first (one-sandwich) test, most of the nonobese subjects ate the sandwich, then went to get more. In the second (three-sandwich) test, they ate one or two, and usually left the third. In contrast, let's look at how the obese subjects behaved. When one sandwich was placed before them, they ate one. When three sandwiches were placed before them, they ate three. They didn't go to the refrigerator for more in either test. The conclusion the testers reached was that obese persons will eat what's available, whether or not they're hungry, while the nonobese persons seem to eat only what they need.

It might be interesting to point out that Dr. Mayer has indicated in his excellent book on obesity (titled *Overweight*) that the words *appetite* and *hunger* are in no way synonymous. Appetite is the complex of pleasant sensations by which one is made aware of the desire for and the anticipation of the eating of *palatable* food. Hunger is the complex of unpleasant sensations felt after a period of deprivation; hunger will cause a man to look for, work for, or actually fight for the food that brings relief from these symptoms.

We need to stop accusing obese people of compulsiveness, of eating to cover up some hidden personal situation. We know that the obese have a defective body image. They suffer from low self-esteem, they're depressed, and they tend to be physically inactive. They need to be prodded into moving, and the younger they start, the better. A sense of physical accomplishment will give them a feeling of well being and this will, in turn, improve their feelings about themselves.

There's one more reason to avoid obesity. If you stop to think about it, I'm sure you'll realize that there's a great deal of prejudice against fat people in our culture. A study done on overweight executives showed that their incomes were lower. I have to admit that I myself would tend to avoid employing a fat person. My prejudices include the impression that fat people are lazy and self-indulgent, and probably won't be on the ball. College admissions are highly influenced by this prejudice.

Another factor to be considered among the causes of obesity is impairment of the mechanism in the brain that regulates food intake. When we sit down to the table to eat, we don't have to stop to figure out exactly how much we'll eat. We go along, eating away. All of a sudden we've had enough. This is because there's a center in the brain, regulating us. This center, called the appestat, is located in the hypothalamus, deep within the brain.

There are numerous biological stats in the body that control our habits after we have set them. They are similar to the thermostats we have in our homes. Here's an example: Most of us don't need an alarm clock to tell us when to get up. Under usual circumstances, we wake up at the same time, almost to the minute, day after day.

The appestat is made up of a feeding center and a satiety center. When the feeding center functions well, it tells us it's time to eat. The satiety center tells us when we have had enough. In the sandwich experiment mentioned above, the satiety center of the obese subjects failed to function compared to those who stopped eating sooner.

An experiment with mice first clarified our concept of the satiety center. The satiety center contains glucoreceptors, which can—and do—inhibit the feeding center. The cells of the satiety center (whose scientific name is *ventromedial hypothalamic nuclei*) have a tremendous affinity for glucose. The existence of these cells was first suspected in cases where the center was destroyed by disease. To knock out the satiety center experimentally, researchers injected into mice a chemical called gold thioglucose, which destroyed the glucose in the cells. Once this area of the brain had been damaged, the mice no longer received signals letting them know when they'd had enough to eat. They kept on eating and eating, and soon became obese.

You can see that all people don't get fat for the same reason. Therapy must be oriented to *cause* if patients are to lose weight and keep it off. The reason so many lose and gain, lose and gain, is that they are all treated the same way, and this doesn't work.

Now for the most important factor of all—physical activity. In Chapter 3 I mentioned the inhabitants of Vilcabamba, a remote village in the Andes Mountains in Ecuador, where Dr. Alexander Leaf found no obese individuals among these people who lived very active lives. He also studied the native population in Hunza, a village in the Karakoram Mountains in Pakistan, where people also lived to be very old and where no fat people are ever seen. These two groups lived on quite different diets, but with equally good results as far as obesity is concerned. The main point was that they were all physically active, virtually to their dying day.

Our problem in the United States is not so much that we eat too much as that we eat more food than is needed for the energy we spend. This situation began when machines started doing the work that used to be done by our arms and legs. The automobile, the washing and drying machines, the elevators and escalators, all cause us to make less physical effort in the course of a day. Yet we eat the same or more (if we can afford it) than if we didn't have these devices.

Why does the body store food instead of merely eliminating what it doesn't need? In primitive society, people did need it. Human beings can store food in the same way as animals that are preparing to go into hibernation for the winter. They need to build up fats off which they can live during the months when they're not able to forage for food. In the same way humans who might not find anything to eat for several days or even weeks ate as much as they could while food was available. When game was scarce, they lived off their fat. The human body is still preparing for that period of famine which no longer comes—at least not in the affluent portions of the United States.

Fat is a very efficient way to store energy. It has nine calories of energy to the gram, while protein and carbohydrate have only four. Since the body can't eliminate fat, storing it is one way of getting it out of the circulation. Unfortunately, if we try to stow away too much, some of the extra is stored in our arteries.

When a member of a track team runs the 100-yard dash, he (or she!) uses chemical substances in his body that release energy rapidly. There's no time to break down anything. He's got to use existing stores of energy that are ready to go. He uses practically no oxygen. The runner takes three or four breaths while he's running that 100 yards. He's used a tremendous burst of energy. Once he's used up his quickly available energy, he begins to break up his fats and they become a major source of fuel. In track events, the dashes are the 100-, the 220-, and the 440-yard. That's as far as a man can go on a spurt of energy. The 880 is known as the 880-yard run.

During a race, adrenal hormones—catecholamines—are secreted. As I'll explain in the next chapter, these hormones elevate the heart rate and blood pressure. Another effect is that fats start to break down, releasing fatty acids. The body then goes through a complicated chemical process, the details of which are far too involved to describe here. Suffice it to say that the end product—the result of oxidation of these fatty acids—serves as a major energy source for muscular contraction. To put it another way, the muscle is able to contract by using as fuel by-products of the breaking down of fat.

If the fight-or-flight reaction—the release of catecholamines and the subsequent release of fatty acids—occurs as a response to emotional stress, and if physical exertion doesn't follow, the muscle doesn't use up those fatty acids. Instead, they circulate in the blood, go back to the liver, and are changed there into particles which are the forerunners of cholesterol. If they were changed back into fats capable of being stored again, all would be as it was before. However, that's not what happens. Because of all these chemical changes, emotion without subsequent physical effort tends to build up atherosclerosis.

Many investigators have done extensive studies on babies. They discovered that many fat babies eat less than thin babies. They also learned that most fat babies were very placid. Inactive was the word for them. The thin babies, on the other hand, were in constant motion. Careful studies showed that the thin infants moved three times as much. The babies' mothers confirmed that this situation held true even before the babies were born. The placid baby had been placid in utero, while the thin one had wiggled and kicked and kept its mother awake at night.

These differences in levels of activity hold true throughout life, even when people seem to be doing the same thing. Some do it with more vigor, with a resulting increase in caloric expenditures. Fat teenagers studied did not eat a lot more than skinny ones; they sometimes ate even less, but they moved around much less. Movies taken showed that even when they were engaging in active exercise—playing volleyball or tennis —they used far less energy. They'd stand and wait for the ball to come to them, while the thin teenager would go tearing after it.

These overweight teenagers are already obese when they start adult life. Just look around any high school or college today. At least one in five is already in trouble.

Some extremely important work is now being done to determine how obesity gets its start. Dr. Jules Hirsch of Rockefeller University and Dr. Jerome L. Knittle of Mount Sinai Hospital

(New York) found that in humans a roughly threefold increase can occur in the number of fat cells found in the body during a baby's first year. This period of rapid growth of fat cells is followed by a much slower but continuous increase. There's another growth spurt between five and six years of age, and another in adolescence. It's believed that cell division probably ceases at some point between puberty and early adulthood.

Dr. Hirsch has developed a special technique for counting fat cells. And Dr. Knittle is currently storing circumcised foreskins in a deep freeze; he plans to compare them with adult tissues, using Dr. Hirsch's technique, when the patient is grown. He is interested in checking to see if he is able to predict in advance whether the patient will be a fat adult. If he's successful, the trend in the future will be toward prevention at an early age.

Once formed, fat cells are not easily destroyed. Restriction of caloric intake can reduce the size of adipose cells, but not the number. That's why it's so important to control the development of obesity in children. I've already pointed out that obese children do not eat more than nonobese kids—unless extra food is forced on them by anxious parents. We suspect that dieting may be harder for people who have a large number of fat cells; the cells may cry out for restoration of the fat they've lost.

The best way to prevent formation of those extra fat cells may be through exercise. Exercise can affect body composition of young, growing humans by lowering or preventing an increase in body fat and by increasing lean tissue. It may be that placid, inactive babies should be made to be more active. Already some pediatricians are prescribing activity periods for infants in preference to letting them just lie still.

The same principles hold for the treatment of obese adults. The watchword is: increase your activity! It is better, in most instances, to eat well and use up more energy. Living on a starvation diet is not healthy, even if one uses vitamin supplements. As Dr. Per-Olof Åstrand of Sweden said, it is healthier to eat more for good nourishment and then become active in the way the human animal was meant to function. That's what we do with our prize animals—proper exercise and proper eating habits.

A pound of fat is worth 3,500 calories. If we want to burn up one pound of fat, activity is the best way. What some people call exercise, others consider the ordinary activity of daily living. For example, a man who weighs 150 pounds, by walking for an hour at a rate of three mph, will burn up 300 calories. The same person, by running or working hard for an hour (if he is in good health) will burn up 800 to 1,000 calories. What he does is decrease the amount of fat in the fat cells, and he does all this without changing his eating habits in any way. If, in addition, he cuts out one dessert, there's another 450 calories (approximately) he won't need to burn up.

There's a widespread belief that increased physical activity is always followed by an increase in appetite. But this is by no means true. In one carefully controlled experiment, grossly overweight male rats were placed in a tank of water where they had no choice but to swim. Over an eighteen-week period, for two hours a day, six days a week, they swam—with a weight attached to each rat's tail, at that. A control group got no exercise. The swimmers took in a total of 8,935 calories, while the sedentary animals consumed 9,985 calories. Many similar studies have all arrived at the same conclusion.

Many of my patients, after they're well launched on a program of prescribed exercises, can't understand why they're actually eating less than before. It's because the satiety center, in animals and humans, does not function properly in inactive people. It's been found that rats confined in small cages eat more than those allowed to run free.

Obesity in and of itself is not going to kill you, but it causes diseases that will do just that. The majority of obese people tend to get high blood pressure. There's a marked increase in their blood volume. When blood volume is increased, people get plethoric—red in the face. You've read about how, before the days of modern medicine, the barber would come and "bleed" a patient. This bleeding did actually help in the cases of some plethoric individuals by reducing the blood volume.

That can be a very useful device. I have had patients who were overweight and full-blooded. Every so often I'd advise them to take themselves to the blood bank to donate a pint of blood. They'd feel much better afterward. It's helpful to reduce excessive blood volume because the extra blood also tends to clot more.

Increased blood volume puts the heart under a strain; it has to work much harder. The obese individual, although he needs more oxygen, will actually get less because his arteries are getting plugged with fat. His heart starts to enlarge from over-work. Eventually the heart can't keep up with the extra work. Too much carbon dioxide remains in the blood. The patient starts to huff and puff at the slightest exertion. You'll notice such patients becoming drowsy and falling asleep at inappropriate times. This reaction is due to carbon-dioxide intoxication. The entire situation is likely to lead to heart failure in extremely overweight patients.

The best time to begin weight control is in early infancy. But you shouldn't throw up your hands with a what's-the-use-it's-too-late-for-me attitude, if your weight is way above where it ought to be. I hope you'll read my chapter on food and eating habits and follow its recommendations. Lose as much weight as you can—safely—as rapidly as possible, with activity, to take some of the extra strain off your heart.

8

Emotions—The Role of Stress in Heart Disease

ACCORDING TO THE BIBLE, when Peter confronted Ananias with the charge, "You have not lied to man but to God," Ananias fell dead. Did he die of humiliation? What about his wife, Sapphira, who died suddenly when told that "the feet of them which have buried thy husband are at the door and shall carry thee out"? Did she die of fear?

Tales of sudden death during moments of strong emotion—fear, rage, grief, humiliation, joy—appear in literature and history as far back as written records exist. Are such deaths merely an interesting part of folklore, or do they continue even today? And if strong emotion does kill, what is the mechanism of death? Dr. George L. Engel of the University of Rochester School of Medicine became interested enough in those questions to start collecting newspaper accounts of death following psychologically traumatic events of one kind or another. After eliminating those deaths that might possibly be attributed to suicide, he wound up with 170 cases. Here is a sampling:

- Ten days after the assassination of President Kennedy, the twenty-seven-year-old Army captain who commanded the ceremonial troops at the President's funeral died, according to newspaper reports, of "cardiac irregularity and acute congestion."

- A fifty-two-year-old man saw his physician frequently during his wife's terminal illness with lung cancer. An examination six months before his wife's death showed no evidence of coronary disease. The day after his wife's funeral the man died suddenly of a massive myocardial infarction.
- A teenage boy on a lark faked a kidnap call to his home. He told his forty-three-year-old father, "If you want to see your son alive, don't call the cops." Four hours later the man died.
- A thirty-five-year-old man accused of robbery told his lawyer, "I'm scared to death!" Then he collapsed and died.
- A fifty-six-year-old man collapsed and died while receiving congratulations for scoring his first hole-in-one.

Few of the newspaper reports collected by Dr. Engel attempted to diagnose the physical cause of death, and Dr. Engel discounts those printed diagnoses which he could not independently confirm. "We can only speculate about the mechanism of death in these cases," he says. "But," he adds, "most would agree that effective cardiac arrest is probably responsible for the deaths of those who collapse and die within minutes. . . ."

Dr. Engel's hypothesis is certainly plausible and logically applicable to many of the cases he collected, and to the anecdotes almost every practicing physician can tell of mysterious sudden death after emotional upset. Human beings, like other animals, have survived in no small measure because of their instinctive ability to run away when afraid or to fight back when angry. This fight-or-flight ability results from a powerful marshaling of the sympathetic nervous system under extreme emotional stress—a marshaling that has come to be called "the sympathetic storm."

The sympathetic nervous system works to accelerate such automatic body processes as heartbeat, respiration rate, and blood pressure. It does this partly by stimulating the adrenals, two glands that sit atop the kidneys. Given an emotional jolt—fear of an impending automobile accident, grief from a death in the family, the rage of an argument, the joy of unexpected good news—the adrenal glands pour into the bloodstream large quantities of hormones called catecholamines. These include epinephrine (adrenalin) and norepinephrine, among others.

The catecholamines prepare the body to muster all its reserves of energy in order to run, or to fight, or to remonstrate with a cruel fate, or to dance for joy. Stored fats and sugars, the food used by cells in producing energy, are released into the bloodstream. The bronchial tubes dilate and respiration rate increases to help the body take in extra quantities of oxygen, needed to metabolize the food in the cells. The pupils of the eyes enlarge to admit more light. Blood pressure rises.

Some of the adrenal secretions also reach the heart to stimulate a faster and more powerful heartbeat. But the heart's role in distributing oxygen is too vital to wait on the progress of hormones through the bloodstream. Dr. Eugene Braunwald, chief of medicine at the Harvard School of Medicine, has recently pointed out that 90 percent of the norepinephrine present in the heart is manufactured right there. The four chambers of the heart are richly endowed with sympathetic nerves leading directly from the brain. Nerve terminals storing norepinephrine are found throughout the heart. When the brain senses a situation demanding a tremendous increase in the work of the heart, it doesn't transmit its message through a relatively slow adrenal interpreter; it says "Go!" directly and in no uncertain terms.

This nervous jolt usually accomplishes its purpose and no more, stimulating the heart into a brief period of superactivity without doing harm. Occasionally, however, especially in hearts weakened by atherosclerosis, the jolt causes ventricular fibrillation, the uncoordinated beating that usually brings sudden death. Or the extra work demanded of the heart may result in a shortage in the heart's own oxygen supply through narrowed coronary arteries and thus in such heart symptoms as angina, or even in myocardial infarction.

If the sympathetic storm can kill, at least it doesn't kill very frequently. We are all survivors of the storm, having many times lived through the pounding heart, sweaty palms, flushed face, and other physical symptoms of strong emotion. We can therefore look forward to the next storm with some confidence, if not pleasure.

Perhaps more dangerous to health than the acute sympathetic storm is the chronic sympathetic drizzle—the daily aggravations and frustrations too minor to bring on an emotional storm but serious enough to keep the catecholamines flowing at a continuously elevated level. The sympathetic drizzle results in that most prevalent and least well understood of modern ailments—nervous tension. And nervous tension in turn brings on a host of physical manifestations, including headache, sleeplessness, stomach upset, colitis, ulcers, asthma—and most important, heart disease.

As long ago as 1910 the gifted Canadian physician Sir William Osler commented about the connection between worry and heart disease among physicians of his acquaintance: "In a group of twenty men [with heart disease], every one of whom I knew personally, the outstanding feature was the incessant treadmill of practice; and yet if hard work—that 'badge of all our tribe'—was alone responsible, would there not be a great many more cases? Every one of these men had an added factor, worry; in not a single case under fifty years of age was this feature absent. . . . Listen to some of the comments which I jotted down of the circumstances connected with the onset of attacks: . . . 'worries in the faculty of Medicine'; 'troubles with the trustees of his institution'; 'law suits'; 'domestic worries.'"

Fifty years after Lord Osler's observations, Dr. Henry I. Russeck, an American researcher, decided to look more closely at the effect of stress on his colleagues. He mailed questionnaires to 4,000 physicians, seeking information on their medical histories. He chose physicians for two reasons. First, because they are trained observers of medical conditions, they are less likely than those in other occupations to be suffering from an illness they don't know about. And, second, they can be divided into specialty groups that experience quite different levels of occupational tension.

His 4,000 questionnaires were divided equally among dermatologists, pathologists, general practitioners, and anesthesiologists. Dr. Russek reasoned (and most of his medical colleagues would probably agree) that dermatologists and pathologists work under much less stress than do general practitioners and anesthesiologists. Dermatologists, or skin specialists, rarely see emergencies or conditions that threaten life. And pathologists rarely see patients at all; they work largely with tissue and microscopes and, Dr. Russeck points out, are "usually in a position to plan or allocate . . . work and commonly enjoy a regularity of working hours." By contrast, general practitioners must cope with "emergency calls by day or night, frequent loss of sleep, and the constant race against time." And anesthesiologists have daily encounters with "potential or real crises in the operating or recovery rooms," are often summoned at unpredictable hours, and must adhere to a rigid time schedule. If occupational stress has anything to do with heart disease, a comparison of these physicians should show it. It did.

Those in the stressful specialties, anesthesiology and general practice, suffered from heart disease at (depending on the age group studied) double or triple the rate of their colleagues in more relaxed modes of practice. A comparison of the two stressful specialties showed additional interesting differences. The G.P.s between the ages of forty and forty-eight suffered heart disease at roughly double the rate of anesthesiologists (6 percent of the G.P.s compared with 2.6 percent of the anesthesiologists). In the next decade, however, the anesthesiologists passed the generalists, and by the time they were in their sixties an extraordinary 30 percent of anesthesiologists had suffered heart disease, compared with 23.3 percent of the G.P.s.

Why did anesthesiologists catch up with and pass general practitioners in the heart-disease derby? "It is well known," Dr. Russeck points out, "that general practitioners tend to lighten their workload on reaching middle age by discontinuing obstetrics, reducing surgical procedures, and curtailing night calls." Indeed, Dr. Russeck adds, the G.P. does so "probably on the advice of his physician." The anesthesiologist, on the other hand, is usually a hospital employee, and therefore not free to taper off in middle age. If anything, Dr. Russeck says, anesthesiologists "are commonly subjected to ever-increasing responsibilities from which there is little or no escape."

At least since the days of Osler, doctors have noted a connection of some sort between nervous tension, or stress, and heart disease. Tension certainly contributes to heart disease indirectly, through other risk factors. For example, some people react to tension by overeating, thereby increasing the likelihood of elevated blood fats and obesity. Tension plays a role in cigarette smoking, an important direct contributor to heart disease, as we shall see in Chapter 9. Tension is widely suspected as the most important cause of chronic high blood pressure, the physical consequences of which are described in Chapter 10. And nervous tension is so physically tiring that the person under constant stress often lacks the energy to exercise during leisure hours.

But the sympathetic drizzle of nervous tension may do a good deal more than merely aggravate other risk factors. In a separate study Dr. Russeck compared a number of risk factors present in 100 coronary patients with the same factors in a control group matched for age and sex. He learned, among other things, that 53 percent of the coronary group ate a high-fat diet, compared with 20 percent of the control group, and that 70 percent of the coronary group smoked thirty or more cigarettes a day, compared with 35 percent of the control group. But the connection between stress and heart disease was even more marked. More than 90 percent of the coronary group worked under severe occupational stress and strain, compared with only 26 percent of the control group.

Those figures would seem to indicate that in addition to contributing to other coronary risk factors, stress plays a *direct* role all its own in the onset of coronary heart disease. Science has not yet pinpointed that role with precision, but recent research projects hint strongly that nervous stress contributes to atherosclerosis, to coronary thrombosis— blood clots in a coronary artery—and to the heart muscle's sensitivity to damage resulting from oxygen shortage.

When you try to measure the physiological effects of nervous tension, you run into problems. Some effects can be attributed to nervous tension alone. And then there are identical effects that are attributable to the physical activity that the tension may have stimulated. It's hard to separate the two.

Two English researchers who wanted to measure the effects of tension met the problem by choosing as their subjects a group of racing car drivers. They reasoned that in few other occupational groups is it possible to pinpoint the specific moments of tension—the race itself—with confidence that during the tense moments the subject is relatively immobile, in this case strapped into the seat of a racing car. The researchers followed their subjects to races in England, Germany, Italy, Spain, and Belgium, taking blood samples immediately before the races and at intervals afterward. They measured the level of catecholamines, the telltale signal of nervous stress, and of fatty acids, triglycerides, and cholesterol.

Predictably, catecholamine levels soared under the stress of driving. Cholesterol levels, however, changed hardly at all, indicating that stress didn't have much to do with the production of that particular component of atherosclerosis. Fatty acids rose to a fairly high level before the race started, remained at a high level until about fifteen minutes after the race, and then subsided to normal in about an hour.

Let's leave our racing drivers for a moment and turn to accountants, people who don't experience much sudden stress but who are subjected to the chronic stress of seasonal pressure. It's been found that, in this occupational group, cholesterol levels do rise slowly during the tax season.

In the racing-driver study, what caught the attention of the researchers, however, was the measurement of triglycerides. When catecholamines were at their highest level and apparently stimulating a rise in fatty acids, triglycerides were at their lowest level. But triglycerides rose to double the normal level by the end of the race and continued to rise after the race, even as fatty acids were subsiding, reaching a peak an hour after the race. Triglycerides were still double the normal level three hours after the race.

The consistent inverse relationship between free fatty acids and triglycerides suggested to the researchers that, under stress, fatty acids were converted into triglycerides, elevating the blood-triglyceride level for long periods of time. Furthermore, the researchers learned, one needn't undergo the stress of an automobile race to trigger that response. "Evidence from electrocardiographic and urine catecholamine studies suggest that these catecholamine levels are probably attained with such mild stimuli as traffic driving, industrial work, and watching films," they reported.

In sum, their research suggests that the stress and strain of everyday life in advanced civilizations may be sufficient to raise the level in the blood of a fat important in atherosclerosis and to keep it raised for long periods of time. It would seem reasonable to speculate that people who experience constant emotional stress are likely to develop atherosclerosis faster than people who don't, other things being equal.

One of the most important catecholamines secreted in large quantities under stress is cortisol, or Cortisone, which stimulates the effective use of sugar during sudden bursts of energy production. But cortisol also depletes the supply of potassium in the heart muscle, and a potassium-short muscle becomes susceptible to rhythm changes or damage caused by oxygen shortage. (That's why astronauts are fed potassium-rich foods while undergoing the rigors of space flight.) Dr. Hans Selye, a leading researcher into the effects of stress, has induced massive heart damage in rats by injecting them with cortisol and then restraining them in a way that made them exceedingly nervous. In rats restrained without cortisol injections, heart damage was rare.

But there's still more to be said about the direct effects of stress. One of the by-products of the sympathetic storm is increased clotting tendency of the blood. Nature not only arranges things so that the body is prepared to fight or run under appropriate provocation, but it also prepares the body to survive wounds. Catecholamines encourage blood platelets, one of the blood components responsible for clotting, to congeal. Sympathetic storms last for only a brief period; the body either finds use for the increased clotting ability during the emergency or it doesn't. After the storm, clotting potential soon returns to normal. But what happens during the steady catecholamine infusion of the sympathetic drizzle? Is it possible that, under constant stress, blood tends to clot even when no wounds make the clot necessary?

A research team headed by Dr. Jacob Haft at Mount Sinai Hospital in New York, not satisfied that the higher oxygen demand under nervous stress was a sufficient explanation for stress-related heart attacks, decided to test the clotting factor in dogs. They treated ten dogs with one drug known to inhibit clotting and another ten dogs with a different drug. A control group of ten dogs was left untreated. Then all the dogs received infusions of epinephrine, the same hormone produced by the adrenal glands, for four hours. A week later the team studied the heart muscles of all the dogs for evidence of necrosis, or death of tissue. All the animals that had not been treated with an anticlotting drug showed necrosis of heart-muscle tissue. Only 30 percent of the treated dogs did. Later studies showed that all the affected dogs "were found to have platelets aggregated in their capillaries."

One cannot draw sweeping conclusions from the experiment, since epinephrine given intravenously may not have the same effect as that secreted by the adrenal glands. But it is certainly "possible," as the researchers say, "that the link between stress and acute myocardial infarction may be via catecholamines . . . leading to the formation of intravascular platelet thrombi that might lodge in an already narrowed coronary."

Or, in plainer language, continual nervous tension may be one *direct* cause of coronary thrombosis.

We all know that people react to stress in different ways. Stress drives some people to great achievement and others to drink. There are those who don't seem to feel stress at all. Although a large percentage of heart-attack victims may have been subjected to stress, a very small percentage of all those subjected to stress suffer heart attacks. Is there something special about those who do suffer stress-related heart attacks?

Some ten years ago, Drs. Ray H. Rosenman and Meyer Friedman of Mount Zion Hospital in San Francisco decided to find out if it was possible to predict from a person's emotional makeup, as expressed in his behavior, whether he was a likely candidate for a heart attack. They were in search of some device for predicting the future because they had already learned, in previous studies, that such traditional risk factors as high blood fats and heavy cigarette smoking, though increasing the likelihood of a heart attack, could not be used as a predictive tool. Too many people who smoked and ate foolishly sailed right on to a healthy old age; too many people who lived like Boy Scouts crumpled nevertheless.

The researchers had noticed certain traits among their own coronary patients, particularly middle-aged and younger ones, that they felt could be considered typical of those who suffered early heart attacks. These traits were what the researchers called Behavior Pattern Type A: "A rather specific combination of personality traits including ambition and competitive drive, aggressiveness, impatience, and a strong sense of time urgency." Most people have some of those traits, the researchers noted, but the Type A man has them "to an enhanced, often excessive, degree. The traits are particularly visible in a person more or less perpetually involved in a struggle in which he is determined to persevere. Sometimes the struggle is with other individuals he feels are out to best him; more often he is 'at war' against time, racing to attain his perhaps unattainable goals before his chance runs out."

To test their hypothesis, the researchers taught lay evaluators what behavioral traits to look for and then had them select from their places of employment a group of men who fit the Type A pattern and a group who, in the view of the selectors, "manifested extreme passivity and lack of drive," a group designated Type B. The two groups were comparable in age (early to mid forties), weight, and dietary habits. A slightly larger percentage of Type A's smoked cigarettes, and those who smoked tended to smoke more than did Type B's (twenty-three cigarettes a day on the average for Type A's, compared with fifteen a day among Type B smokers). Type A men also had higher cholesterol levels, on the average, and slightly shorter blood-clotting times.

Of eighty-three Type A men examined, twenty-three

showed either cardiac symptoms or electrocardiographic evidence of clinical coronary disease. Only three of eighty-three Type B men showed evidence of heart disease.

But perhaps, one may argue, the Type A men were subject to more-stressful situations than the Type B men. Maybe it's the stress that made them Type A in the first place. Or maybe Type A's gravitate toward stressful occupations and personal lives. At the time of their first study of Type A and Type B men, Drs. Rosenman and Friedman also studied a third group, neither Type A nor Type B, but under severe stress. This group was made up of forty-six blind men whose physical handicap resulted in "chronic anxiety and insecurity . . . emotions not characteristic of Type A men." Only two of them showed any evidence of heart disease.

It's not the *fact* of stress that counts, the researchers concluded, but the individual's *particular reaction* to stress.

In the next phase of their research, the two investigators prepared a questionnaire designed to elicit angry and aggressive feelings, in order to evaluate the degree of a subject's drive and ambition, and, above all, his sense of time urgency. (Sample questions: Do you often have the feeling that time passes much too fast for you to accomplish what needs doing each day? Are you impatient when someone does a job slowly that you could do faster? Do you often step in and do it yourself?)

Trained interviewers used the questionnaire to interview 3,500 subjects. Responses were tape recorded. So as not to make prejudgments about the possibility of heart disease from observations about a subject's obesity or smoking habits, Drs. Rosenman and Friedman did not personally meet any of the subjects. Working only from the taped answers to the questionnaire and from the intensity and emotional overtone of the answers, the doctors divided the subjects into types. They found that they could classify roughly 10 percent as extreme Type A's and another 10 percent as extreme Type B's. About half of the remainder fell into a moderate Type A classification and the other half into moderate Type B.

Here is how the researchers describe an extreme Type A: "The Type A person is invariably punctual and greatly annoyed if kept waiting; he rarely finds time to indulge in hobbies, and when he does, he makes them as competitive as his vocation. He dislikes helping at home in routine jobs because he feels that his time can be spent more profitably. He walks rapidly, eats rapidly, and rarely remains long at the dinner table. He often tries to do several things at once and carries a second line of thought if he can possibly manage it." The Type A person tends to answer questions emphatically, often explosively. His voice is loud and at times even hostile in tone. "In his impatience, he anticipates what others will say . . . and frequently interrupts to answer questions before they are fully asked." If he had a coat of arms, "it would feature a clenched fist wearing a stopwatch."

Once typed, all subjects were examined. The Type A's stood out from the beginning. Preexisting coronary disease was found in 113 of the subjects. More than 70 percent of those 113 had previously been characterized as Type A's.

Eight and one-half years after they had been typed, some 250 of the original 3,500 men had experienced coronary heart disease. The rate among Type A's was 13.2 per thousand per year; among Type B's, 5.9. To be sure, coronary risk factors other than the characteristic reaction to stress played an important role in the likelihood of heart disease. For example, placid Type B's with blood cholesterol levels of 260 or higher suffered heart disease at precisely the same rate as all Type A's. But that same risk factor superimposed on a Type A behavior pattern proved downright disastrous. In Type A's with high cholesterol levels the heart disease rate soared from 13.2 to 21.8 per thousand per year.

There's no question that most Type A's who are satisfied

with their achievements get along fine. Reduction of drive and ambition isn't going to benefit the Type A; it's the reduction of *frustrations* that counts. A study by the Metropolitan Life Insurance Company showed that the top executives of leading corporations have a longer life expectancy than other American men. That study concluded that "work satisfaction, together with public recognition of accomplishments, is an important determinant of health and longevity."

To sum up, emotional stress may be second in importance only to manner of eating as a factor contributing to heart disease, and some would put stress first. It contributes to overeating, cigarette smoking, and high blood pressure. And it may play a direct role in atherosclerosis, coronary thrombosis, and embolism. Emotional stress that triggers extreme competitiveness, aggressiveness, ambition, and impatience is particularly dangerous.

Unfortunately, too few people, doctors included, are fully aware of the severe consequences of stress, perhaps because there's no easy way to deal with its causes. The nagging boss won't just go away, and neither will the nagging wife. Traffic will continue to crawl, as will waiters. Planes will be late coming and going. The stock market will go down about as often as it goes up. Children will become less perfect with each passing year. Movies will become more pornographic, unless you happen to like pornography, in which case they won't.

Yet ordinary life stresses are not necessarily beyond individual control. To quote again from that Metropolitan Life study, you can "thrive on stressful situations by harnessing tensions for productive use." Unfortunately, we can't all be presidents of large, successful corporations. But we can cut down on frustrations and increase the amount of fulfillment in our lives. If you don't like your job, find one you like better. You can divorce a spouse who makes you miserable.

You can beat traffic jams by getting to work early—or late. You needn't go to restaurants if slow service makes your blood boil, and if you can't stand investment losses you can buy U.S. Savings bonds. You can expect less of your children, and you can stop going to movies—or start.

In short, you can take control of some of the important stresses in your life *before* a heart attack makes it a matter of survival. After his heart attack, Monte sold his interest in the business, which he considered the main source of his worries. He's an employee now, not a part owner. He no longer gives much of a damn about what happens before he gets in at nine or after he leaves at five. Having come close to death, he is trying to find different values in life. He wishes he had changed his life style sooner.

Changes in life style may strike some as psychologically naive. It can be argued that you behave and react the way you do because of a particular roll of the genetic dice modified by a lifetime of environmental conditioning. No superficial changes in life style at the age of forty or fifty will change your psychological makeup. The uptight Type A raging at the impossibility of accomplishing twelve hours of work in an eight-hour day can tell his boss to shove it, sell the house with the big mortgage, and pack his family off to a commune—where he will proceed to rage at the impossibility of growing four crops of tomatoes during one summer.

Drs. Rosenman and Friedman, however, believe that a Type A person can both simplify his life in ways that reduce stress and change his characteristic reaction to stress. They emphasize that their research did not deal with a "coronary-prone personality" but with "an overt behavior pattern which results from the interaction of a given individual with his specific environment."

Dr. Friedman long ago classified himself as a Type A (in his youth his friends called him "Cannonball"), and true to type he suffered a heart attack six years ago. As a result of both his professional experience as a research cardiologist and his personal experience as a heart patient, he offers this advice to his fellow Type A's: Force yourself to slow down internally. If you catch yourself thinking about more than one thing at a time, stop. Such polyphasic thinking is a great mental strain. Never interrupt what someone else is saying; force yourself to wait, no matter how boring or obvious the conversation may appear. Read books that can't be skimmed, that force you to concentrate—philosophy, economics textbooks, involved novels. Eat food slowly, trying to savor every bite.

Repeated practice in slowing down the daily tasks of thinking, conversing, reading, and eating can develop new habits of behavior, he believes.

Beyond that, Dr. Friedman recommends that Type A's build more relaxation into their lives. Find a place at home where you can have total privacy for some part of every day, away from family, television, and animals. Avoid people who bother you, as much as possible. Perhaps you can't really avoid your boss, or the guy who works at the next desk, but you can certainly get out of a lunch date with someone you've known for years and don't really like. Figure out ways to avoid time pressure. If you find yourself rushing through your morning routine to get to work on time, set the alarm clock half an hour earlier and dress more slowly. Simplify your schedule; avoid doing too much in one day.

In short, Dr. Friedman gives the same advice doctors have long given their patients: Take it easy. I know from my own experience that there's no better advice I can give any heart patient or potential heart patient. Nor, I regret to say, is there any piece of advice less likely to be followed. If you can't take it easy, for whatever reason, then control of all the other risk factors mentioned in this book becomes increasingly urgent.

Let's look once more at the numbers developed in the

study of Type A's and Type B's. During any given ten-year period 132 out of every 1,000 Type A's are likely to develop coronary heart disease. If a Type A can't reduce stress or change his reaction to stress, that's the chance he takes. Add a cigarette habit, however, and the chance grows to 175 in 1,000. Add a high cholesterol level and it's 218 in 1,000. Add chronically high blood pressure and it's 227 in 1,000.

The numbers speak for themselves. Heart disease is largely environmental in origin. You can avoid it to the extent that you are willing and able to control your personal environment.

9

Cigarettes–
The Addiction That Kills

THE 1964 SURGEON GENERAL'S REPORT
showed that the total death rate was 70 percent higher for
smokers than for nonsmokers. The required notice on every
package of cigarettes and on every cigarette advertisement
reads: "Warning! Smoking is dangerous to your health."

If you still smoke cigarettes, it's not an act of bravado. The
fact is that a large number of smokers are drug-habituated—
habituated to the drug nicotine in almost the same way other
addicts are addicted to heroin. The main difference is that
nicotine addicts are killing themselves faster and more surely
than heroin addicts.

Every cigarette costs a man six minutes of life. A twenty-five-
year-old nonsmoker has 48.6 more years to live. If he smokes
two packs a day, he has only 40.3 more years.

Smoking contributes importantly to a whole host of illnesses,
from the common cold to lung cancer. But its contribution to
heart disease, and particularly to sudden death from a heart
attack, is most dramatic. Dr. Jeremiah Stamler, professor of
medicine at Northwestern University's medical school, says
the incidence of sudden death in a first heart attack is 20
percent in heavy smokers.

Dr. Stamler has plenty of company in the statistical gloom-
and-doom department. Dr. David M. Spain, head of pathology

at Brookdale Hospital in Brooklyn, did an intensive study of the information on autopsies of 189 men who had died suddenly from coronary heart disease. He discovered that for every sudden death of a nonsmoker under the age of 50, there were 16 sudden deaths in those who smoked more than a pack a day. Recently, Dr. Daniel Horn, director of the National Clearing House for Smoking and Health, reported that studies showed that two-thirds of the deaths from heart attack in men between 45 and 49 are chiefly caused by cigarette smoking.

Doctors don't depend simply on mortality statistics about smokers versus nonsmokers when they conclude that smoking isn't one of your healthier habits. We've also studied the anatomy and physiology of what happens in the human body when you smoke.

Smoking one to two cigarettes causes an increase in heart rate of fifteen to twenty-five beats per minute. It causes a rise in blood pressure, both systolic (10 to 20 millimeters) and diastolic (5 to 15 millimeters). Besides affecting heart rate and blood pressure, those one or two cigarettes also cause a decrease in the flow of blood through the fingers and toes. We can actually measure a drop in temperature there. Blood is warm. So when less of it circulates through the small capillaries in the extremities, they become cooler. When I find a patient with cold feet in a warm room, I can safely conclude that his circulation is poor. Thus, smoking makes for poor circulation, thereby aggravating peripheral vascular disease.

To understand how smoking causes all these reactions in the human body, refer back to the preceding chapter, in which we talked about the effects of the catecholamines—the hormones secreted by the adrenal glands in times of stress. We've already discussed how the catecholamines stimulate the liver to release stored fats and sugars into the blood, cause the heart to beat harder and faster, blood pressure to rise, and the respiration rate to increase, so the body can take on extra oxygen, and so on.

Well, stress isn't the only trigger for the catecholamines. Nicotine stimulates the adrenal glands of modern men and women just as efficiently as a hungry tiger tickled your ancestors' nervous systems. Your liver and your heart have no way of knowing that no tiger is after you. They only know how to respond to the message of the catecholamines.

Nicotine exorbitantly increases the oxygen consumption of the heart muscle, and, in the extremities, it causes constriction of the small blood vessels. It causes the blood pressure to rise (we'll be talking about that in the next chapter) and it also increases the ability of the blood to coagulate. Or, to put this in less scientific terminology, it actually "makes the blood stickier."

If you inhale—and most cigarette smokers do—the harmful effect of nicotine is much greater than if you don't inhale. To understand the reason for this you need to know something about the anatomy of the lung.

The air you breathe passes down through the trachea, into the main bronchi (the branching tubes of the trachea), thence into the smaller bronchioles, and finally into the alveolor spaces—microscopic sacs where the oxygen from the air passes into the capillaries. If you could spread all the alveoli in your lungs out flat, you would have an area equivalent to half a tennis court. When you inhale, this whole enormous area absorbs nicotine from that puff of smoke. If, however, you don't inhale, but only take the smoke into your mouth, only the comparatively small mouth area absorbs nicotine.

Nicotine's effect on the adrenal glands is just one of the physical changes that occur when you smoke a cigarette. Let's talk about the carbon monoxide in tobacco smoke. Nicotine is the addictive agent in tobacco smoke; its physical effects are what the smoker craves. But carbon monoxide may be the bigger killer.

Tobacco smoke contains up to 4 percent by volume of carbon monoxide, so you inhale a little carbon monoxide with each puff on your cigarette. Unfortunately, the hemoglobin in your blood has much greater affinity for carbon monoxide than it does for oxygen, and therein lies a problem, as we'll see shortly.

Hemoglobin is the chemical in your red blood cells that carries oxygen to your tissues. In the tissues, the hemoglobin unloads the oxygen it's been carrying and picks up the carbon dioxide that is the waste product of the cell's metabolism. This waste product is carried back to the lungs, where it's released as you exhale.

Now comes the problem. Hemoglobin's affinity for carbon monoxide is somewhat over 200 times greater than for oxygen. If there is any carbon monoxide around, the red cells will pick it up in preference to oxygen. Therefore the presence of even small amounts of carbon monoxide reduces the capacity of the blood to transport oxygen.

A study found that subjects who smoked ten to twelve cigarettes a day had 4.9 percent carbon-monoxide hemoglobin; the percentage rose to 6.3 percent in those who smoked fifteen to twenty-five cigarettes a day; smokers of thirty to forty cigarettes a day showed a percentage of a whopping 9.3 percent. (Other researchers have found it as much as 20 percent.) If they then quit smoking entirely, it took at least twenty-four hours for the carbon-monoxide content of the blood to return to normal.

You get no symptoms from less than 10 percent concentration of carbon monoxide in the blood—not unless you run for a bus, play a little handball, go in for any kind of physical exertion. If you do that, you'll notice it. How? You'll have to huff and puff, gasping in an effort to get needed oxygen to your tissues.

Dr. Poul Astrup's group of Danish researchers studied 1,000 factory workers, of whom fifty-eight were heavy smokers. Every one of the fifty-eight was found to have atherosclerosis of the coronary arteries, and every one of them had a high level of carbon monoxide in his blood. The levels varied with the depth and duration of inhaling. Cigar smokers who inhale were in the worst shape of all, with levels as high as 25 percent of carbon monoxide in the blood.

Dr. Astrup found that smoking makes the blood vessels more permeable. Fat appeared to flow through the blood-vessel walls; some of this increased flow of fat was deposited in the walls. And there you have it—atherosclerosis.

At the University of Pennsylvania's medical school, Dr. Arthur F. Whereat has spent a good deal of time studying the mechanism of the atherosclerotic process. He found that the arterial wall is an active participant in this business of the manufacturing of fats. The cells that make up the wall contain very small bodies, called *mitochondria*, within their protoplasm. It is within these microscopic structures that the fatty acids are manufactured.

The cells of the arterial wall are in a constant process of building up fats and breaking them down. Carbon monoxide (and other respiratory inhibitors in our environment) seems to poison the cells, changing the way fats are manufactured, so that the amount of fat they produce is increased.

It is the problem of carbon monoxide that dooms efforts to make smoking safe by developing a nonnicotine cigarette. An interesting series of experiments was carried out by Dr. Wilbert S. Aronow of the V.A. hospital in Long Beach, California. He had heart patients smoke lettuce-leaf cigarettes. He worked with a group of patients with the type of heart disease known as angina pectoris, a disease I described in Chapter 2.

Dr. Aronow had these angina patients smoke ordinary cigarettes, cigarettes low in nicotine, and cigarettes made out of lettuce leaves instead of tobacco. (Lettuce contains no nicotine whatsoever.) Even smoking lettuce-leaf cigarettes caused an increase in blood carbon-monoxide levels and brought pain to angina patients during exercise.

Each patient was studied on two occasions after smoking

eight of those lettuce-leaf travesties in a four-hour period and on two occasions after a twelve-hour period of no smoking. During each study period, the patients were exercised on a bicycle ergometer, a stationary bike on which the subject pedals against a measurable load. On the mornings following a twelve-hour period without smoking, a patient could pedal for 110 seconds without getting pain. But after he'd smoked, he could only go for 83 seconds.

The problem, you see, is that carbon monoxide is the product of incomplete combustion. It's produced by burning lettuce leaves, burning tobacco, burning gasoline—burning almost anything.

We get carbon monoxide into our lungs in many ways other than by smoking. One of the classic cases is that of a patient who had suffered from angina, but who took his doctor's advice, changed his way of life, and was rewarded. He stopped having those pains. Then, one afternoon toward the end of an all-day out-of-town meeting, he suddenly developed severe chest pain. The reason? The meeting had been held next door to a garage. All day the patient had been breathing in exhaust fumes loaded with carbon monoxide. The result was the same as if he'd started smoking again.

Travel on expressways during rush hour is a real health hazard, particularly to cardiac patients. In order to make sure that the attacks of angina that heart patients reported were due to carbon monoxide, and not to the stress of driving in heavy traffic, Dr. Aronow did a carefully controlled study. His test patients were driven in a station wagon over similar routes on two different days during morning rush hour. The doctor chose a Los Angeles County expressway for the experiment. The first morning, the men breathed that famous California air through an open window. Blood samples were taken right before the trip, immediately afterward, and, finally, two hours later. A few weeks later these same men took the same trip, the only difference being that they wore plastic headgear (like astronauts), through which they received purified air from a tank.

Dr. Aronow found that the levels of carbon monoxide rose significantly after the first drive, but not after the second, when the men were breathing purified air. He also proved that the angina effects brought on by exercise began significantly sooner after the first drive.

But the air in heavy traffic contains only about seventy-five parts per million (ppm) of carbon monoxide. Cigarette smoke contains about 400 ppm of carbon monoxide. So think how much worse smoking must be. There's been so much written and said about air pollution, I don't want to go into it any further, here. But I can't resist reminding you that, when you fill the air in a small conference room with cigarette smoke, the amount of carbon monoxide in that room will rapidly exceed the amount that is a legally acceptable exposure in industry.

Even if you refuse to worry about what your smoking is doing to your own tissues, you should give some thought to its effect on your family. Whenever they're in the room with you, your children are breathing in the carbon monoxide from your smoke and reducing the amount of oxygen to their tissues. If one of your children has asthma, your smoking increases the child's symptoms. Specialists at the Mayo Clinic advised parents of asthmatic children never to smoke in the child's bedroom, in the car when the child is along, or in any room where the child is sitting.

Speaking of children, there is strong evidence that pregnant women who smoke are taking significant chances with the health of their unborn babies. A report published by the British Public Health Service in 1972 showed that smoking mothers had a stillbirth rate 30 percent higher than nonsmokers and an infant death rate for the first few days after birth 26 percent higher. There's a probability that this heightened risk to the unborn infant can be eliminated if the mother gives up smoking by the fourth month of pregnancy.

There's no question that women smokers bear children with a lower average birthweight. Every study that's been done confirms this.

Throughout this discussion I've been talking about carbon monoxide and blaming it for interfering with the blood's normal hemoglobin-oxygen transport system. Dr. Robert W. Eliot, a cardiologist in Omaha, Nebraska, who has been directing an investigation at V.A. hospitals, found that carbon monoxide causes the red blood cells to hold onto their oxygen, instead of releasing it as they should. For some unknown reason, this is particularly true in women. This lessening of the ability of oxygen to leave the red cells and get into the tissues occurs in the heart, and also in the legs and feet. Doctors are now beginning to suspect that it must affect the brain, too. They're always finding something new to worry about.

Dr. Eliot's work has also turned up the fact that even after all the carbon monoxide has been removed from smokers' blood, the red cells' ability to pick up oxygen continues to be impaired. Dr. Eliot suspects that some other substance, still unidentified, remains in the smokers' blood as long as the habit continues. He wonders whether blood donors who smoke are really doing a sick patient much of a favor when they bestow their tainted blood plasma on him.

Blood banks, which have enough trouble as it is, keeping their stocks up, aren't eager to start rejecting smokers' blood. As future studies turn up more facts, they may have to do it nonetheless.

Dr. Eliot has done a good many studies on women who smoke heavily and found that many of them were having heart attacks or angina even though they have perfectly normal coronary arteries. In these patients the release of oxygen into the tissues had been impaired.

Fortunately, there's no need to despair. The body has a remarkable ability to recover, if you give it a chance. Perhaps you've read about the famous experiments carried out by Dr.

Oscar Auerbach and his smoking beagles. After the dogs had been smoking for a number of months, microscopic studies of their lungs showed what we doctors call *metaplasia*—that's a premalignant cellular picture. If the dogs continued to smoke heavily, this stage soon progressed into malignancy. If, however, the dogs were taken off cigarettes, the abnormal cells disappeared within a year.

The heart, too, is able to stage a complete recovery, in time —if you give it the opportunity. The 1964 Surgeon General's report, to which I referred at the beginning of this chapter, shows that a patient who stays off cigarettes for five to ten years reduces his risk of death almost to that of one who has never smoked. In several studies, mortality ratios of ex-smokers have been compared with those of smokers and of nonsmokers. The figures show a 41 percent reduction in mortality risk for ex-smokers. The longer the discontinuance, the greater the reduction in risk.

Now let's see what happened to patients who recovered from a heart attack and then gave up smoking. These patients had just about half as many fatalities from repeat coronaries as smokers who stayed with the habit. Dr. Risteard Mulcahy of St. Vincent's Hospital in Dublin, president of the Irish Heart Foundation, conducted a study of ex-smokers and found among them a five-year mortality rate of 18 percent as compared to 34.5 percent among those who kept right on smoking. Figures on the patients who continued to smoke showed that 40 percent of the deaths occurred within the first twelve months after that initial attack, as compared to 20 percent in the groups that reduced or stopped smoking. It's hard to believe, but *none* of the non-smokers died during the five-year period of the study.

Okay, okay! you say, irritably. You've convinced me. I should stop smoking. But suppose for the moment that I'm able to do it. The people I know who quit proceeded to gain a lot of weight. What about that?

You're right. Many—though certainly not all—of those who stop smoking do indeed gain some weight. There are several reasons for this. Remember that old slogan "Reach for a Lucky instead of a sweet"? It works in reverse, too. But overeating is not the *only* reason for weight gain. Doctors think that a change takes place in the body's metabolism. One study showed that the basal metabolism did change. The metabolic rate became lower—showed a decreased basal oxygen consumption. The patients in this study hadn't changed their eating habits or the amount of physical activity. They gained weight because they weren't burning up their tissues as rapidly.

Naturally, you don't want to get fat. But you don't need to be concerned about it. If you're very careful for the first six months—watch your diet, get more exercise—your metabolism will change back. What you do have to worry about is just how you're going to go about quitting.

Nobody is going to tell you it's an easy thing to do.

Rockefeller University's Dr. Vincent P. Dole, a leading authority on heroin addiction, says, "Cigarette smoking is a true addiction. The confirmed smoker acts under a compulsion which is quite comparable to that of the heroin user."

At Synanon, a therapeutic community for heroin addicts, cigarettes had been supplied to residents along with food and clothing. Most of the residents were heavy smokers; the tab came to almost $200,000 a year. Charles A. Dederich, founder and head of Synanon, told a *New York Times* reporter, "We decided to ban smoking and to make it a community crime, punishable by shaved heads or eventual expulsion." Dederich reported reactions that included depression, irritability, and weight gains of from 7 to 30 pounds. Residents said that, unlike most drugs, whose withdrawal symptoms last a week at most, withdrawal symptoms for tobacco last at least six months. They found it was much easier to quit heroin than cigarettes.

Many research studies have been done to determine what

causes this addiction. One of the best was conducted at the University of Michigan medical school. The subjects of the experiment spent six hours a day for fifteen consecutive days in a soundproof, air-conditioned isolation booth, with a needle in an arm vein. They could read or smoke or do whatever else they chose. On some days saltwater was fed into the vein through the needle; on other days a nicotine solution was fed in. It's important to explain here that none of the subjects knew that the experiment had anything to do with smoking or nicotine. They did know there was an ashtray handy, so they could smoke if they wanted to.

On days when saltwater was injected, the subjects smoked an average of 10.1 cigarettes per six-hour session. On nicotine-injection days, they smoked only 7.3 cigarettes—and left longer butts. That's important, because a longer butt means a significant reduction in nicotine consumption; the cigarette itself acts as a filter. Much of the nicotine in the early puffs of smoke stays in the cigarette. It only reaches the smoker in the later puffs.

In another experiment the subjects, smokers all, lay in bed with continuous IVs (intravenous solutions) of nicotine dripping into their veins. As long as the nicotine was dripping, their tendency to reach for a cigarette was way down. Their addiction was apparently satisfied. Discontinue the nicotine in the IV and they'd soon light up.

I can confirm these experiments from my own experience. When I was at military school, all the kids smoked. We were twelve and thirteen years old and felt that smoking made us big shots. In the spring we went to camp for two weeks of military maneuvers. Being under the direct observation of our instructors, we didn't dare smoke, so we all chewed tobacco. You could follow our platoon by the spit! Chewing tobacco satisfied our nicotine addiction because the body doesn't care in what form it gets the drug. This fact accounts for the recent increase in the use of snuff, which also satisfies the nicotine addiction.

It's easy enough to break the habit of reaching for a ciga-rette. That takes about a week. Breaking the addiction takes much longer. If you're one of those people who can't break it, you may have to substitute a less-irritating way of satisfying the addiction, such as cigar smoking—without inhaling, of course.

The fact that nicotine is an addictive drug is not widely known. It should be. Young people should be warned. Those who never begin to smoke will not have to cope with breaking the habit.

I quit smoking the day the 1964 Surgeon General's report came out. My motivation was, very simply, that I didn't see how I could tell a patient to stop smoking while I myself was smoking. He'd think I was a pretty weak-willed character.

At least 95 percent of my patients who've had heart attacks have given up smoking, but a heart attack is a lousy way to get your motivation! If you find that you simply can't quit cold, taper off by switching to a pipe—but don't inhale it. If you find you're inhaling the pipe, get the lousiest, cheapest cigar you can find. The old Italian stogie is the kind I mean. If you inhale even that, then chew tobacco. If that doesn't work, try one of the organized groups, such as SmokEnders, Smoke Watchers, etc.

A very important part of your motivation is your spouse. If he or she goes on puffing smoke in your face, you'll never make it. Your partner will have to quit, too. But be sure you do your share by emptying your smelly ashtray frequently if you're tapering off with a cigar, and by spraying the air—carefully. Incidentally, we're beginning to worry about the harmful effects of those aerosol sprays.

Once you've won the battle, you'll be amazed at how much better you'll feel. Your immunity to viral infections will in-crease, your blood pressure will drop—and so will your medi-cal bills. It's an established fact: Families that smoke have higher medical bills and more chronic illness.

10

Blood Pressure–
The Silent Disease

HYPERTENSION, OTHERWISE KNOWN as high blood pressure, has been called "the silent disease" because it so often fails to display any unique symptoms. People with high blood pressure can go along for twenty years or more with no idea that they're harboring a dangerous condition. Then, suddenly, everything starts to fail at once—including the blood vessels.

Before I get much further into high blood pressure, let's make sure you understand just what blood pressure is. By its rhythmic pumping, your heart builds up pressure in the arteries. This pressure moves the blood through the arteries, into the tissues. When the heart muscle contracts, it pushes the blood through the arteries, speeding up its flow. When the heart muscle relaxes between pushes, the blood doesn't stop flowing entirely, of course. It just slows down. That's the reason we use two numbers to designate blood pressure. If your doctor writes on your chart the figures 120/80, the first number indicates the greater pressure (the systolic pressure) exerted during the heart's contraction; the second number shows the lowest pressure (the diastolic), which occurs during the rest period between contractions. (The device used to measure blood pressure contains a column of mercury as the measuring stick. So a blood pressure reading of, say, 120 means that the blood pressure equals the pressure exerted by 120 millimeters of mercury.)

Doctors used to believe that "normal" blood pressure should be computed by adding the patient's age to the number 100. They thought that normal systolic pressure for a man of fifty would be 150. At age sixty, 160 would be satisfactory pressure. That idea has long since been discarded. While it's true that in the United States many people's blood pressure does rise ten points for every ten years of aging, that is neither normal nor desirable—it's merely another indicator of our abnormal and unhealthy way of life.

What, then, is normal blood pressure? Believe it or not, no one knows for sure. But certain facts are known. Follow-up studies done over the past fifty years by insurance companies on their policy holders indicate that people with blood pressures higher than 140/90 have increased mortality rates. Most physicians now use this figure of 140/90 as the highest acceptable level at which blood pressure can be considered normal. Anyone with blood pressure higher than that should be under medical treatment.

Insurance-company figures also show that the higher the blood pressure, the higher the death rate climbs. On the average, people with blood pressures below 110/70 live the longest. In that study of the villagers of Vilcabamba done by Dr. Alexander Leaf, seven of those aged 100 or more averaged blood pressures of 135/64.

Temporary increases in blood pressure are, of course, perfectly normal. In Chapter 8 we talked about how the body reacts to stress. When you are startled by a sudden loud noise, or frightened by an alarming situation—a mugger approaches you, or your baby stands up in his high chair and is in imminent danger of pitching out onto his head—you get what Dr. Hans Selye has called an "alarm reaction." Instantly, your body responds to the emergency: The sympathetic nervous system stimulates the adrenal glands to pour catecholamines into your system. They in turn cause a rise in pulse and blood pressure, and an increase in blood sugar; the heart, the lungs, and the skeletal muscles all go on an alert. The result is that the circulation gets moving very rapidly. The blood is thus able to carry fuel—in the form of oxygen and glucose—to the muscles so that they can react swiftly. Within seconds, thirty to forty times more blood will be coursing through your leg arteries than before you were aware of danger. With the extra strength and energy at your disposal, you take off in a burst of speed, away from that mugger—or you lunge forward to catch the baby before it hits the floor.

That's one kind of temporary rise in blood pressure. Another is one on which every participant in active sports relies heavily. In a baseball game, if the man at bat has to duck a wild pitch, it's the rise in blood pressure and pulse rate (along with quick reflexes) that enables him to move fast enough to avoid getting beaned.

Dr. Selye, who is the director of the Institute of Experimental Medicine at the University of Montreal, also refers to this reaction to stress as the body's "call to arms." It's a necessary reaction for survival. However, once the immediate emergency is over, all systems should return to normal. If they don't, you get a condition we call *chronic stress.*

Epidemics of high blood pressure have been reported among soldiers fighting in World War II in the desert of Libya. Over 30 percent of these men had blood pressures of 180 or higher.

Chronic stress can be produced experimentally. In one study, men were given mental arithmetic problems to work out, and while they were doing so, a ticking metronome annoyed and distracted them. They responded with a typical alarm reaction, including elevation of arterial pressure, increased heart rate, and increased flow of blood to the muscles.

Dr. J. Alan Herd of Harvard and his group subjected squirrel monkeys to a set of completely controlled and unfamiliar circumstances. The monkeys were placed in chairs in a very small room and required to respond, by pressing a lever, to flashes of light. The wrong response resulted in an electric shock. After a few months Dr. Herd's monkeys developed high blood pressure. Their pressure reached its highest level while they were in the isolation booths and dropped sharply as soon as they were removed from the chambers. The monkeys' blood pressure then gradually rose again. Directly before the next session, it took a sudden upward spurt. Thus, animals actually learned to raise their blood pressure in response to the lights. Eventually their blood pressure became fixed at a high level and didn't go down between sessions.

One more very interesting fact was learned from these experiments. Only nine of the eleven experimental monkeys developed hypertension under pressure. Dr. Herd concluded that a genetic factor must be involved. Some individuals are more susceptible than others to stress in their environment.

Dr. Herd points out an analogy with the human experience. He says most of us have to confine ourselves to a small space in an office or on an assembly line, curtailing our gregariousness and responding to cues—the alarm clock, the phone, the factory whistle, and so on. If our responses are incorrect, we don't get electric shocks, but we do get punished. The boss gets angry; the raise doesn't come through. How many of us, like those monkeys, respond to such stress with temporary increases in blood pressure that eventually become permanent increases?

Like so many factors connected with heart disease, high blood pressure appears to be another product of so-called civilization. Dr. Ian Prior, director of the Epidemiology Unit at the Wellington Hospital in New Zealand, conducted a series of studies to find out the effects of civilization on blood pressure. For his study, he and his group, which included not only physicians but also nutritionists, sociologists, and anthropologists, studied different groups of Maori peoples (all Polynesians). Dr.

Prior found that the farther from civilization he got, the lower was the incidence of high blood pressure (and of high cholesterol as well). Among the most primitive, the Pukapuka people, one man in fifty had high blood pressure. Among the Maoris of New Zealand, one man in five had high blood pressure.

In Pukapuka—a coral atoll in the Cook Islands—they live a simple life. With a cash income of about $36 a year, they can't afford the products of civilization. They live largely on a basic diet of fish, taro (a starchy root eaten throughout the tropics), and coconuts. There's no salt added to the food.

Probably the most important physical way in which the human animal induces his blood pressure to go up is by eating sodium chloride—or salt. There's an ancient Chinese saying: "If too much salt is used in food, the pulse hardens." Interestingly enough, the saying is true.

Northeastern Japan is notorious for the high salt intake among its population—and for the high rate of cerebrovascular disease. The local farmers and their families ate a traditional diet of heavily salted preserved foods, pickles, soy sauce, and so on. They ingested up to 20 grams—about 5 teaspoons—of salt a day. That's a lot of salt. In 1957 the authorities introduced meals relatively low in salt into the schools of Akita, a city in the area. They started an educational campaign to try to get adults to join their children in eating foods prepared with much less salt. In 1971 Professor Naosuke Sasaki of the Hirosaki University School of Medicine reported an initial decline in the systolic blood pressure of children converted to the low-salt diet. He also reported that the expected "normal" rise in pressure of about 10 millimeters of mercury per ten years had failed to occur.

Why does salt raise the blood pressure? It's a matter of simple physics. Water tends to flow into a highly concentrated salt solution. A high salt content in the blood draws fluid, thus increasing the volume of blood in the circulation. Salt also gets into the walls of the arteries, which proceed to swell. Naturally, the swelling causes narrowing of the vessel; thus, the blood pressure must increase in order to push the same amount of blood through the narrowed vessel.

For millions of years, wrote Dr. Eors Bajusz, all mammals have had a problem conserving salt. The ability to conserve salt used to be a survival trait. The body never developed any kind of mechanism for getting rid of excess salt because there never was any excess. Now that modern diet provides too much salt, we eliminate it too slowly. All the body can do is call for more water in order to keep the extra salt in solution. Thirst is the signal. Salt makes you drink more. When you do, the total volume of liquid goes up. Then the pump has to pump at a higher pressure to move the extra liquid around. Not being designed to pump such a large volume of fluid, the pump has to overwork.

A group of doctors from the National Heart and Lung Institute found that people with high blood pressure consumed four times as much salt as a control group with normal pressure. These hypertensives also took in twice the amount of fluid.

Many experiments have been conducted to find out exactly what salt does to your blood pressure. One group of investigators from Brookhaven, New York, took baby rats from a strain of rat ancestors who were unusually prone to hypertension and fed them a diet of strained human baby food, which is highly salted. A control group of baby rats ate a low-salt diet. The controls grew up strong and husky, while almost all the rats fed from jars of human baby food developed hypertension. You can induce high blood pressure at a very early age.

More than 100 years ago—in 1836, to be precise—Dr. Richard Bright found that people with certain kinds of diseased kidneys suffered from high blood pressure. He believed that these patients' problem was primarily a kidney disease. It wasn't until around 1911 that doctors began to realize that the high blood pressure was affecting the kidney, instead of the other way around. In one of the landmark contributions of the century, Dr. Harry Goldblatt succeeded in inducing hypertension experimentally. He put a hemostat, or surgical clamp, on an animal's renal artery (the main artery that carries blood to the kidney). He didn't close it off completely, just partially. As the blood flow became more and more obstructed, the animal's blood pressure rose.

Well, what have all these experiments taught doctors about the causes of high blood pressure? Frankly, not all we want to know. We believe that stress contributes to hypertension. We believe that there may be a genetic tendency toward hypertension. And we believe that a high-salt diet has something to do with the condition.

But what do we know for sure? We do know that certain specific and curable physical conditions account for a small number of cases of high blood pressure, probably fewer than 10 percent of all hypertension cases. Those specific physical problems are atherosclerosis of the renal arteries (the arteries leading to the kidneys) and a rare type of tumor of the adrenal gland. Before I go on to discuss the vast majority of hypertension cases, I'd better explain these two unusual physical conditions and how they cause a few cases of high blood pressure.

All blood flows through the kidneys, just as all blood flows through the heart. The kidneys remove the waste products picked up from the cells when the blood delivered its freight of oxygen. Sometimes atherosclerosis, the same mushy deposits that occur on the walls of the coronary arteries, narrows the walls of the arteries leading to the kidneys. What happens is exactly the same as what happens when you squeeze a water hose. Pressure must rise to force the blood through the narrowed opening. Thus, hypertension.

Now about the possibility of a tumor on the adrenal gland. (It's called Conn's Syndrome, after Dr. J. W. Conn, who first described it.) If the tumor exists, it produces a hormone called aldosterone. That in turn triggers a whole series of chemical reactions that would take a book to describe and a doctorate in chemistry to understand. But the end result of those reactions is that the kidney fails to excrete salt. Your body retains more salt than it should. And too much salt, as you already know, causes high blood pressure. Researchers are also investigating other theories about why the kidneys might fail to eliminate salt, but Conn's Syndrome is one theory that's been proved.

If your doctor should find that you are suffering from hypertension, he may run you through a battery of x-ray examinations and other types of blood tests such as renin, angiotensin, etc. to see if the cause is physical. If it is, the chances of a surgical cure are excellent. Many physicians will not do many tests, because, the chances are greater than nine out of ten that they will find no physical reason for your hypertension. The doctor will then pronounce the following diagnosis: "Essential hypertension." That's what most people with high blood pressure have. But what does "essential hypertension" mean? It simply means "high blood pressure of unknown cause." In effect, you have hypertension and we don't know why.

While it would certainly help to know the cause, it helps too to know what damage hypertension brings—and it also helps to know that even though we don't know what causes most cases of hypertension, we do know how to control them and thus steer clear of the damage.

Constant high blood pressure causes blood vessels to lose elasticity and also forces fats into the arterial wall, thus increasing atherosclerosis. Myocardial infarction or stroke (brain hemorrhage) are a couple of the many complications to be expected. Elevated blood pressure also increases the risk of kidney failure and angina.

In addition to its effect on blood vessels, high blood pressure forces the heart to pump too hard. Eventually the heart starts to give out—or fail, as doctors say. In heart failure, the muscle simply lacks the strength to push the blood around. The result is swelling in the legs and congestion in the lungs. Thus the term "congestive heart failure." A heart muscle weakened by years of being forced to pump harder than it should is less likely to survive a heart attack than is a normal muscle.

Among patients with elevated blood pressure, the proportion who died within a month after suffering their first myocardial infarction is twice that of normotensives (doctorese for patients with normal blood pressure). Hypertensives also have double the usual risk of a second heart attack and more than five times the risk of dying from it.

But believe it or not, from the *doctor's* point of view, high blood pressure is a *minor* problem in most instances—if only the patient is treated. Few illnesses are easier to detect and control than high blood pressure. (There are exceptions; it can be serious, but these cases are unusual.)

Years ago, when I found that one of my patients had hypertension, about all I could do was prescribe a little phenobarbital and tell him or her to take it easy. Now we have a wide variety of tests to separate the minority of cases with a physical origin from the majority of unknown origin. The physical problems can be cured surgically. More important, most cases of essential hypertension, the mysterious silent disease, can be *completely* controlled under a doctor's care. The doctor can prescribe the right drugs for each patient's particular problems. We have drugs called diuretics, which help to lower salt content and get rid of excess water. We have medicines that can quiet the nervous system. We have drugs that can neutralize the action of the catecholamines. Of course, the amount of salt we eat is the easiest of all the factors to control. We should be paying the most attention to that. Exercise also helps to lower blood pressure, so good physical fitness is also helpful.

It is estimated that there are more than 20 million people in this country whose blood pressure is elevated above 140/90. Almost 30 percent of the individuals whose blood pressure is checked in surveys of the general population are in this category.

Essential hypertension is usually incurable. But all that means is that we don't know how to lower high blood pressure without permanent treatment. So what? With the proper permanent combinations of diet and drugs, essential hypertension is controllable. That means, to put it simply, that anyone with high blood pressure who gets on a medically controlled treatment regimen will *not have high blood pressure* so long as he stays on it. In effect, as long as he takes treatment, he's as good as cured.

11

Exercise–Why Without It
You Are Endangered

IT TAKES TWO MEN to run one of London's dou-
ble-decker buses. One man drives. The other, the conductor,
roams upstairs and down, back and forth, collecting fares and
assisting people boarding and debarking. The driver sits all
day. The conductor keeps moving. That's one important difference between them. Another important difference is the rate
at which they suffer heart attacks.

In a famous study reported in *Lancet*, the British medical
journal, some twenty years ago, researchers noted that London
bus drivers suffered nearly twice as many myocardial infarctions as conductors, and more than twice as many drivers died
of heart attacks as did conductors. That was the first really
strong association of physical activity with a reduced incidence
of heart attack and of inactivity with an increased incidence of
heart attack. But, as the researchers themselves recognized, it
was an *association*, not proof that physical activity—exercise
—protects against heart attacks.

Perhaps other factors accounted for the driver's relative sus-
ceptibility to heart attacks. While the conductors were getting
their exercise, for example, the drivers were steering the big
vehicles through the clogged London streets. Anyone who has
ever driven in city traffic knows the kind of aggravation those
drivers must have felt. Perhaps the stress of driving played an

important role in the statistics. Or perhaps there were subtle genetic differences between drivers and conductors. When the London transit authorities hired conductors they turned down tall men because tall men would have to spend the day uncomfortably stooped within the confined space of a bus. No such height restrictions were applied to drivers.

I mention those caveats merely to point out that a single study, no matter how interesting and suggestive, is insufficient reason for large numbers of men to abandon their easy chairs and start exercising. The evidence linking inactivity with an increased risk of heart attack, however, isn't based on one study alone. The study of London bus drivers and conductors sparked a whole series of similar population studies around the world. With few exceptions, they confirm the main thrust of the London study.

In North Dakota, for example, it was found that farmers suffered roughly half as many heart attacks as nonfarmers. In general, it's probably fair to say that farmers are physically more active than nonfarmers, so the difference in heart-attack rate between those groups provided another clue linking inactivity with heart attacks. But aren't there other differences between farmers and nonfarmers besides their degree of physical activity? Indeed there are, and perhaps some other factors contributed to the statistics. But the North Dakota study turned up still another clue. One of the important differences among the farmers themselves was that some owned tractors and other labor-saving devices and some didn't. As a result, some worked a lot harder than others. Those farmers who worked especially hard, who put in at least one hour of heavy physical labor a day, suffered heart attacks not at half the rate of inactive men but at only one-fifth the rate.

A similar study of people living on kibbutzim, or cooperative farms, in Israel, where almost the only environmental differences between people are in their assigned tasks, showed that those in active jobs—farmers, laborers, and so on—suffered about one-third as many heart attacks as office workers and others in sedentary occupations.

One of the most ambitious controlled-population studies was undertaken by Dr. Frederick J. Stare, chairman of the Department of Nutrition at the Harvard School of Public Health. With the help of researchers at Trinity College School of Medicine in Dublin, Dr. Stare compared the health over a ten-year period of 600 Irish-born men who had come to Boston with that of their brothers who had remained in Ireland. None of the men studied was more than five years younger or older than his brother.

The prevalence of death from heart disease about doubled after ten years' residence in the United States, Dr. Stare reported. Why? One couldn't lay the blame on the American diet this time. In fact, the brothers who remained in Ireland ate an average of about 500 more calories per day, and those calories included far more butter and eggs, foods known to raise blood-cholesterol levels. Yet the average blood cholesterol of the brothers in Ireland was 13 percent lower than that of those in America. Further, despite their higher intake of calories, the Irish brothers weighed 8 to 10 percent less than the Americans, and, reported Dr. Stare, they showed "essentially no fatness—all were lean and muscular."

The main difference between the brothers, Dr. Stare concluded, was that those in Ireland "worked harder physically— there were fewer modern gadgets at work, and when they went calling, most of them went by foot or on bikes."

Study followed study. Postal clerks suffered more heart attacks than mailmen who walked their rounds; railroad clerks died of heart attacks at twice the rate of switchmen and maintenance workers. The studies tend to become repetitive. Their collective message is clear, though: Exercise reduces your chances of heart attack.

Perhaps just as important, exercise greatly improves your chances of living through a heart attack. Here are the statistics:

Among inactive men suffering their first heart attack, one in five dies; among active men suffering their first heart attack, only one in twenty dies.

To understand how exercise protects against heart attack, let's recall what a heart attack is. Basically, a heart attack is a shortage of oxygen in the heart muscle severe enough to damage muscle tissue. The shortage occurs when atherosclerosis interferes with or stops the supply of blood through the coronary arteries, or when the heart demands more oxygen than the diseased arteries can supply.

Not too many years ago, doctors advised their heart patients to rest, rest, and then rest some more. The advice was logical enough. Activity makes the heart work hard and demand more oxygen. Since a heart patient was known to have diseased arteries, activity carried the risk of excessive demand and thus of another heart attack. These days, however, physicians often urge their heart patients not to rest but to exercise —mildly at first and then more actively. In effect, heart patients are advised to go into training much as an athlete does. Reason: Physical training changes the supply-and-demand equation in the patient's favor.

Here's how:

1. *Exercise makes the heart a more efficient pump.* All muscles need oxygen to produce energy. An efficient muscle needs a lot less oxygen for a given unit of work than an inefficient muscle needs, just as an efficient automobile engine needs less gas per mile than an inefficient engine.

The effect of training on the heart muscle's efficiency is easy to measure. Ask an average, presumably healthy, patient of forty who's out of shape to walk a mile at a fair pace—let's say in twenty minutes. Then take his or her pulse. You'd probably find the heart pumping at the rate of 110 to 120 beats per minute. Now train the patient by making sure he or she walks that same mile regularly, say three or four times a week, for two months. You'd then find that the pulse rate after the mile had dropped to about 100 beats per minute. The workload has remained the same, but the heart is meeting it with less effort. It has become more efficient.

Several things have happened to permit the heart to work less hard during that walk. The leg muscles have grown more efficient; they extract from the red blood cells a larger proportion of the oxygen in circulation; and there's more oxygen available because exercise also increases the total volume of blood in the arterial system. With the leg muscles using oxygen more efficiently, the heart needn't circulate the blood as fast as it did two months before. It can beat more slowly.

At the same time, the heart itself has become more powerful. With each beat, it squeezes out a larger volume of blood than it did before. That increase in stroke volume, as it's called, also allows the heart to beat more slowly and thus reduces the heart's own demand for oxygen.

2. *Exercise increases the number and size of blood vessels.* The circulatory system can be visualized as a marsh fed by a network of arteries and arterioles and drained by veins and venules. Between the arterial system and the venous system lies the marsh, made up of connecting open channels called capillaries. That's where the action is. The cells absorb oxygen through the capillaries in exchange for carbon dioxide, the waste product of the combustion process known as energy.

Physical training forces the whole circulatory system to expand. Some latent capillaries open up, improving the flow of blood in the marsh. Other capillaries grow into arterioles, small arteries. Arteries themselves become wider.

The process has benefits throughout the body (which is a contributory factor in the more efficient use of oxygen), but it is especially significant in the heart, where an interruption in the oxygen supply threatens life. A physically conditioned man is less likely to suffer a heart attack than a deconditioned man because his coronary arteries are wider and therefore less apt to clog up with atherosclerotic mush.

If he does suffer a heart attack, he's more likely to survive. Some researchers credit his improved chances to the extra blood vessels that have developed in the heart—the coronary collateral vascularization, as it's known medically. Perhaps the extra blood vessels compensate fully or partly for the blocked blood vessel. Others credit the trained man's survival to his heart's efficiency—to the possibility that the undamaged heart muscle is more likely to work well enough to sustain life than would be the case in an untrained man. Perhaps the complete answer is a combination of the two factors. No matter what the precise mechanism, it's clear that exercise is what brings it into play.

3. *Exercise increases the amount of oxygen the body can actually use.* It is possible to determine the oxygen used by having a subject pedal an exercise bicycle while breathing into a large bag. The oxygen the subject has consumed is determined at the end of the test by measuring the contents of the bag. Not long ago, researchers tested nine men between the ages of thirty-two and fifty-nine who were sedentary not by choice but because they had been blind for at least ten years. Repeated measurements over three months showed that their oxygen uptake was relatively constant and uniformly low, averaging 24 milliliters of oxygen per kilogram of weight per minute (which is the way scientists measure these things).

Then the men were trained with daily workouts on the exercise bicycle three times a week for fifteen weeks. At the end of that period they were tested again. Their oxygen uptake had increased by an average of 19 percent.

What does this mean? If you looked at microscopic photographs of the cells of their leg muscles taken before and after exercise, you would notice an increase in the number and size of mitochondria—the part of muscle cells that stores energy. Those cells are now ready to produce much more energy on demand than they could before physical training. They will therefore require less work of the heart, another factor that allows a trained man's heart to beat more slowly than an untrained man's at a given level of exercise.

4. *Exercise may help reduce blood clots* that lead to coronary thrombosis and embolism. Blood tends to clot more readily immediately after exercise. That's a natural adaptive process. Human beings in nature didn't exercise for the fun of it. They exercised to hunt their food—or other humans. Their chances of injury were therefore higher than those of today's marathon runner, or even of a professional football player. The faster their blood clotted, the better their chances for survival. At the same time, however, exercise increases the body's production of a substance called *fibrinolysin,* which dissolves blood clots.

Thus the natural response to exercise is increased clotting ability to stem the loss of blood in case of injury and at the same time increased ability to dissolve a clot once the danger has passed. Some believe that this characteristic response to exercise helps account for some of the protection a conditioned body enjoys against heart attacks. The increased tendency of the blood to clot, it is reasoned, is too temporary for clots to form in coronary arteries. But the increased production of fibrinolysin may well counter the tendency of blood to clot around atherosclerotic deposits.

5. *Exercise helps you control your weight.* We have discussed the relationship between obesity and heart attacks. Exercise, despite some propaganda to the contrary, plays a significant role in weight reduction. As noted earlier, you gain weight sure as night follows day when you take in more calories than you spend in activity; you lose weight sure as day follows night when you spend more calories in activity than you take in in your food.

Weight-reduction diets typically fail because the dieter grows too hungry to stay with it. You can eat more and satisfy your hunger without gaining weight simply by burning up the calories in exercise. The table on page 123 shows the calories used in typical physical activities. Note that a brisk half-hour walk can use up about 200 calories. That's enough to permit the hungry dieter an extra 3½ slices of bread, or a cup of cooked rice, or ½ cup of potato salad—without gaining an ounce.

We've already debunked the notion that your appetite increases when you exercise. In Chapter 7, we talked about the appestat, the regulatory mechanism in the brain that tends to adjust appetite to physical activity, so that you eat about as many calories as you spend in physical activity. A sedentary life, a life virtually free of exercise or hard physical work, throws the appestat out of whack. If you do little or no exercise, your appetite will not decline enough so that your caloric intake matches your caloric outgo. You will gain weight. So exercise is absolutely essential in controlling weight.

Furthermore, if you play your physiological cards right, you can use exercise to beat the regulatory mechanism temporarily while trying to lose weight. When you exercise, blood rushes to your extremities—the legs when you walk or run, for example, and the arms when you swim—to supply the increased demand for oxygen. Blood rushes away from those parts of the body that need the oxygen less—namely, the digestive system. With less oxygen in the digestive system, activity there falls off. Appetite is temporarily suppressed. The dieter's strategy, then, should be to exercise vigorously just before exposing himself to the temptations of a big meal. He will arrive at the table a little more sweaty but a little less hungry. By the time his appetite catches up with his energy expenditure, dinner will be over.

A good deal remains to be learned about the many ways in which exercise benefits the heart. For example, some researchers report that exercise keeps blood cholesterol and triglycerides low. The Irish brothers are a case in point. Among other population groups with low cholesterol levels, by American standards, are the Bedouins who drive camels across the Sahara desert. Unlike the Japanese, or the Vilcabambans, or the West Malaysian aborigines, the Bedouin camel drivers eat saturated fat in quantities that would be disastrous for Americans. On their treks, camel butter becomes the center of their diet. Why doesn't the high-fat diet result in high blood-cholesterol levels? It's widely believed that the Bedouins simply walk it off.

Exercise may also play a role in controlling high blood pressure, according to several reports. Much more research will be needed to confirm that interesting possibility. Still, the known physiological effects of exercise on the heart are sufficiently beneficial to make a planned program of exercise an obvious part of any preventive health regimen.

The benefits of exercise don't end with the observable physical effects. The subjective, psychological effect of exercise should not be overlooked. Many people who have begun to exercise and who have stayed with it until exercise has become a habit report an increased sense of well-being and a greater tolerance for the psychic assaults of everyday life. They are less nervous, they sleep better, they are less open to the damaging physical effect of stress discussed in Chapter 8.

Many people who exercise soon learn how much fun they can have while protecting the heart. They may take up tennis, or ride a bicycle long distances, or get back to one of the team sports like basketball or touch football that provided so much pleasure in their younger days. Once that happens, the physical effects of smoking, described in Chapter 9, hit home. One can intellectually accept the idea of severely damaged lungs from smoking, but it's not until you run out of breath halfway through your first set of tennis that you're likely to really do something about the habit. Lots of patients who have tried in vain to give up cigarettes finally report success when motivated by the desire to play winning tennis or to get involved in pick-up basketball games on the weekend—or just to take a brisk walk on a fall day without wheezing and coughing.

CALORIES USED IN SOME PHYSICAL ACTIVITIES

		CALORIES PER MINUTE	CALORIES PER HOUR	NUMBER OF MINUTES TO BURN UP	
				CHOCOLATE CAKE 450 CAL	TWO SLICES OF BREAD 120 CAL
WALKING					
Walking	2.5 mph	3.5	210	129	34
Walking	3.0 mph	5.0	300	60	24
Walking	3.75 mph	5.6	335	80	21
Walking	4.0 mph	6.2	372	73	19
Jogging	6.0 mph	11.0	660	41	11
SWIMMING					
Swimming Crawl, Slow		6.5	390	69	18
Swimming Crawl, Fast		12.5	750	36	10
Swimming Sidestroke		9.0	540	50	13
BICYCLING					
Bicycling	5.5 mph	4.5	270	100	27
Bicycling	10 mph	5.3	318	85	23
Bicycling	13 mph	11.0	660	41	11
SPORTS					
Volleyball		3.5[1]	210	129	34
Bowling		4.4[2]	264	102	27
Golf with Caddy		6.2[3]	372	73	19
Ice Skating		6.2	372	73	19
Table Tennis		6.5	390	69	18
Golf, Pulling Cart		7.0[4]	420	64	17
Tennis, Doubles		7.1	426	63	17
Canoeing		8.3	498	54	14
Skiing, Downhill		9.9[5]	594	45	12
Tennis, Singles		11.5	690	39	10

1. Too low if played at all vigorously.
2. The usual sociable game is somewhat lower.
3. Playing a fast twosome.
4. With a heavy bag.
5. Doing turns as an expert does.

Convinced? Ready to rush out and run a mile? Don't.

Exercise can also kill you if you go at it the wrong way. And not all exercise is equally beneficial. In the next two chapters we'll discuss how and how much to exercise, and how to make exercise a safe and beneficial part of your way of life.

12

The Exercise Test–Who Needs One Before Working Out?

THE AMERICAN HEART ASSOCIATION has a special committee on exercise. Recently, this committee told doctors that there was some epidemiologic evidence supporting the view that maintenance of a high activity level is in itself an effective preventative against the development of coronary heart disease. Translated into simple English, this statement means that evidence obtained from a study of actual heart disease gives support to the theory that active exercise helps in preventing heart disease. I have already described some of the evidence in previous chapters.

If you test Americans under thirty-five, you don't find many abnormal tests; after that age, you begin to find more and more abnormals. Therefore, I recommend that, for safety's sake, it's probably best that, before starting any exercise program, any middle-aged American (age thirty-five or older) should have an exercise stress test, as should younger people with a family history of heart disease.

A resting electrocardiograph tells your doctor only where you have been. A cardiograph recorded under the stress of exercise shows him where you are going—what your heart can be expected to do over a period of time. Sometimes that resting cardiograph will be normal, while the tracing made under stress shows early signs of trouble to come. Nearly 40 percent of those who die suddenly from coronary artery disease or who suffer acute myocardial infarctions have had no previous symptoms to warn of impending disaster.

In this country, the treadmill is the most popular machine in use for exercise testing; in Europe, a bicycle exercise machine called an ergometer (work meter) is more commonly used. Both are equally reliable. The treadmill routine most doctors prefer for testing patients over thirty-five is to have the patient walk at a steady two miles per hour while raising the grade every two minutes. Younger persons are started at three miles per hour and may go even faster later in the test.

If a bicycle ergometer is used, the patient starts pedaling on the bike, with more tension put on the pedals every two minutes or so. As the tension increases, the patient has to push harder. Meanwhile, the doctor watches the electrocardiograph, looking for abnormalities that may start to appear. There may be changes indicating that the heart muscle is suffering from insufficient oxygen.

The harder you exercise, the higher your pulse rate goes—but only up to a point. The younger you are, the faster your pulse can go. If you've ever held a feverish small baby very closely, you must have felt its heart going bang! bang! bang! However, as you get older, the ability of the pulse rate to go more rapidly diminishes. After a certain point, no matter what you do, your pulse rate won't go any higher. You may run even faster or jump even higher, but your pulse rate simply cannot go faster. That point is known as "maximal rate for age."

When we do an exercise stress test, we doctors have the option of testing the patient to his maximal capacity, or we may decide that testing to some lower point is good enough. Theoretically, in order to find out precisely how the heart performs under severe stress, we should test the patient under increasing stress until he is completely exhausted and can go no further. However, it is only in university settings or in teaching hospitals that patients are tested in this way. We get just about as much information without pushing the patient to such an extreme degree. Now and then maximal rates may come up with some extra findings, but usually it is neither necessary nor advisable.

For ordinary purposes (testing in the doctor's offices or community hospitals) it is felt that submaximal testing is sufficient. Patients are tested to 85 percent of maximal pulse rate for their age. Turn to the exercise chart on page 150. Let's take, as a sample, a person who is thirty years of age; the theoretical maximal rate would be about 194. The same person's maximal rate at the age of sixty would be about 160. This person's submaximal rate at age thirty would be 165; at age sixty it would be 135.

Here is the procedure you can expect when you go for exercise testing. First of all, you'll be weighed. Next, a series of electrodes will be strapped to your chest with wires leading to an electrocardiograph machine. In some laboratories the EKG may be transmitted by radio. A blood-pressure cuff will be wrapped around your arm so the pressure can be checked at frequent intervals. You will now be asked to start exercising. As you do so, the doctor will be watching your cardiograph and checking your blood pressure constantly. As the test proceeds, the doctor takes the blood pressure at frequent intervals and watches the cardiograph. Should there be changes indicative of myocardial anoxia (not enough oxygen reaching the heart muscle), they will show up on the portion of the EKG tracing known as the S-T segment. Should this portion of the tracing drop below the base line, it's a sign that the heart muscle is crying out for oxygen. Should the heartbeat become dangerously irregular, should the patient complain of severe chest pain, or should the blood pressure drop, the doctor immediately terminates the test. (The blood pressure must actually rise at each step during the test; the more work you are doing, the higher your blood pressure goes.) If none of these situations occurs, the doctor knows that the heart is able to perform adequately under that particular physical stress. If it fails to perform as it should, the doctor knows at exactly what level it started acting abnormally.

After testing, an actual prescription of exercise can be written. The doctor will have you exercise at a pulse rate that is between 70 percent and 85 percent of maximal rate for your age. If you don't exercise to about 70 percent of the maximal rate, you probably won't be doing enough to do you much good. On the other hand, if you exercise between 70 percent and 85 percent, you'll improve your physical condition. After some weeks of training, your pulse rate gets slower in relationship to the load. Your blood pressure will tend not to rise as much as it did before training. For instance, if you're retested on the bicycle ergometer early in your training period, you might get a pulse rate of 130; a few weeks later the same load might show a pulse rate of only 120 and your blood pressure would be lower. The pulse rates of trained athletes are quite slow, both at rest and during the various loads.

The doctor can perform the test so that the result comes out either in Mets or in calories of effort. One Met is the amount of oxygen an individual uses when at rest. A calorie is the amount of energy required to raise one gram of water one degree centigrade. A calorie is a unit of heat. That's why we measure various foods in terms of calories. What we're measuring is the number of units of energy produced by that food when we "burn it up."

Let me give you some examples of how all this works out in practical terms. Suppose you are walking on a treadmill at a rate of 2 mph. If your doctor has set the grade at 7 percent, you're using up about 4 Mets' worth of effort. Four Mets is the approximate equivalent of doing bricklaying, wheeling a wheelbarrow with a 100-pound load, or of cleaning windows. In terms of recreational activities, 4 Mets is the equivalent of taking a 3-mph walk, or riding a bicycle at 6 mph, or pitching horseshoes, or playing volleyball, or playing golf (with a caddy carrying your clubs). Now suppose your doctor advances the treadmill to a grade of 10½ percent, which is 5 Mets. Five Mets is the equivalent of doing masonry work, paperhanging, or light carpentry. It's the recreational equivalent of walking 3½ mph, cycling at 8 mph, playing table tennis, dancing the foxtrot, raking leaves (if you call that recreation), or carrying a reasonable number of golf clubs as you play around the course. If you reached 10 Mets, you'd be doing the equivalent of shoveling sand, running 6 mph, or skiing.

When a bicycle ergometer is used, test results appear in calories of effort. On the ergometer, we test in terms either of footpounds/minute or kilogram meters/minute or calories/minute. Our 4-Met result is equivalent to approximately 5 calories. Five Mets is about 6 calories, and 10 Mets is 11 to 12 calories. Putting it in graphic, easily understood terms, the doctor may say to you, "I just tested you at the equivalent of walking the way you used to do it in the Army: Hut! Two! Three! Four!" If you will turn to the chart on page 130, you will find a list of activities, and you can see for yourself how one activity compares with another in effort expended.

Now then, how about sex? How much energy does it require? Much less than you probably think. Dr. Herman Hellerstein of Cleveland found that it requires 7½ or 8 calories, or 6 to 7 Mets of energy, with pulse rates that average 117 to 120 per minute; that's approximately the equivalent of walking up two to three flights of stairs. If you can do that without feeling exhausted, there should be no problem. However, that statement holds true only for sexual relations with wives! In extramarital situations the death rate is quite high. "Motel death," it's been called. In Japan a researcher named Ueno reported that he had found 34 out of 5,559 sudden deaths in which sex seemed to play a part. Half of these occurred during extramarital relationships—undoubtedly due to nervous tension. The blood pressure and pulse rate go much higher, making intercourse much more hazardous.

ENERGY REQUIREMENTS OF COMMON ACTIVITIES
(measured in calories per minute)
1.2 calories = 1 MET

OCCUPATION			
Watch repairing	1.6	Chopping trees	12.0
Typing	1.8	Lifting more than 100 lbs.	16.0
Driving tractor	1.9	**SELF CARE**	
Painting, sitting	2.0	Resting, supine	1.0
Gardening, light	2.1	Sitting	1.2
Armature winding	2.2	Standing, relaxed	1.4
Cobbling	2.2	Feeding self, sitting	1.4
Hammering nails	2.4	Conversation	1.4
Using hand tools	2.5	Dressing, undressing	2.3
Radio assembly	2.7	Propelling wheelchair	2.4
Driving car or truck	2.8	Washing hands, face, standing	2.5
Sewing at machine	2.9	Walking slowly, 1 mile	
Upholstering	3.0	in 24 min.	3.5
Sawing, power hand	3.1	Dressing, washing, shaving	3.8
Planing soft wood	3.4	Showering	4.2
Sweeping or raking	3.4	Walking downstairs	5.2
Mowing lawn, power	3.8	Walking (military),	
Bricklaying	4.0	1 mile in 16 min.	5.6
Plastering	4.0	Walking, level, icy street	5.6
Tractor plowing	4.2	Walking moderately fast,	
Assembly-line work	4.5	1 mile in 15 min.	6.2
Pumping tire	5.0	Walking uphill, 5% slope	7.2
Horse plowing	5.9	Ambulation, braces and crutches	8.0
Sawing soft wood	6.3	Walking fast, 1 mile in 12.5 min.	8.0
Carrying 50 lbs.	6.7	Climbing, descending,	
Carpentry	6.8	2 flights stairs/min.	8.5
Pushing wheelbarrow	7.0	Walking level, 2.5 in. snow	10.7
Pulling, light	7.0	Walking uphill, 10% slope	13.0
Sawing hard wood	7.3	**EXERCISES**	
Mowing lawn by hand	7.7	Walking slowly,	
Digging	8.0	1 mile in 24 min.	3.5
Felling tree	8.0	Cycling, 5.5 mph,	
Shoveling earth	8.5	1 mile in 11 min.	4.5
Ascending stairs, 17 lb. load	9.0	Straight leg raising	4.8
Shoveling sand	9.0	Swimming, 20 yds/min.	5.0
Splitting wood	9.0	Walking briskly,	
Planing hard wood	9.1	1 mile in 20 min.	5.0
Pulling hard	10.0	Walking (military),	
Tending furnace	10.2	1 mile in 16 min.	5.6
Climbing ladder	10.4	Rowing, alone	6.0
Chopping with ax, pick or		Swimming, 30 yds./min.	7.0
sledgehammer	10.8	Walking fast,	
		1 mile in 12.5 min.	8.0

Climbing, descending, 2 flights of stairs/min.	8.5
Master two-step test	8.5
Deep knee bends, 30/min.	9.0
Push-ups, 30/min.	9.0
Running, 1 mile in 11 min.	11.0
Cycling, 13 mph, 1 mile in 4.5 min.	11.0
Walking, 5 mph, 1 mile in 12 min.	11.0
Running, 1 mile in 9 min.	14.0
Running, 1 mile in 7.5 min.	17.0

HOUSEWORK

Hand sewing	1.4
Cooking, standing	1.6
Painting	1.6
Sweeping floors, light	1.7
Machine sewing	1.8
Polishing furniture	2.4
Light ironing, standing	2.7
Scrubbing, standing	2.9
Peeling potatoes	2.9
Laundering, light	3.0
Dusting	3.1
Vacuum cleaning	3.2
Kneading dough	3.3
Scrubbing floors	3.6
Cleaning windows	3.7
Mowing lawn, power	3.8
Filling washing machine	4.1
House painting	4.1
Making beds	4.1
Heavy ironing	4.2
Mopping	4.2
Waxing floors	4.2
Wringing by hand	4.4
Hanging wash	4.5
Beating carpets	4.9
Washing floors	5.3
Carrying 20 lbs.	5.3
Putting wash thru hand wringer	5.7
Carrying 50 lbs.	6.7
Shoveling snow, moderately wet, 10/min.	11.4

RECREATIONAL

Embroidering	1.2
Rug hooking, sitting	1.3
Knitting	1.5
Typing	1.8
Playing cards	2.0
Painting, sitting	2.0
Chisel carving	2.0
Working in garden, light	2.1
Power sanding	2.2
Playing piano	2.5
Driving car	2.8
Golf, putting	3.0
Horseback riding, slow	3.0
Volleyball	3.5
Walking slowly, 1 mile in 24 min.	3.5
Golf, using irons	3.7
Throwing	4.0
Bowling	4.4
Cycling, 1 mile in 11 min.	4.5
Golf, using woods	5.0
Swimming 20 yds./min.	5.0
Cycling, 10 mph, 1 mile in 6 min.	5.3
Dancing foxtrot	5.5
Gardening, moderate	5.6
Golf, walking with caddy	6.2
Ice skating	6.2
Sawing soft wood	6.3
Table tennis	6.5
Washing, waxing car	6.5
Dancing rumba	7.0
Golf, pulling cart	7.0
Golf, carrying bag	7.0
Tennis, doubles	7.1
Sawing hard wood	7.3
Trotting horse	8.0
Canoeing	8.3
Spading	8.6
Skiing, tow, downhill	9.9
Squash	10.2
Cycling, 13 mph, 1 mile in 4.5 min.	11.0
Swimming, crawl, fast	11.5
Tennis, singles	11.5
Running 1 mile in 8 min.	11.7
Skiing, cross-country	12.0

These values are only very approximate, but they do give a relationship between one activity and another. Thus, this chart is to be used as a guide only.

Let's take a look at some of the practical results of exercise testing. In 1968 Dr. Richard Call, medical director of the Union Oil Company, did an exercise test as part of the annual physical examination for 400 male executives, aged twenty-four to sixty-four. None of these men had any symptoms of heart disease. He used a treadmill for his routine "roadtest" for heart performance. One out of every seven men he tested showed signs of deficient circulation of blood to the heart muscle. None of the men in their twenties had any difficulty. As for the men in their thirties, 5 percent already showed some signs of lack of oxygen. In the forty-five- to fifty-year-old group, 15 percent had trouble. The percentage rose to 29 percent among men aged fifty to sixty, and to 55 percent for those in their early sixties. Naturally, if any of those who had positive reactions went in for strenuous exercise, it could have been dangerous.

Dr. Call plans to follow up the 13.6 percent of the men who showed evidence of insufficient cardiac circulation; he has, of course, recommended programs designed to prevent the occurrence of a heart attack.

Now I want to tell you about the work of the late Dr. Samuel Bellet, director of cardiology at Philadelphia General Hospital. Dr. Bellet did a study of 795 employes of the Bell Telephone Company, all of whom were apparently healthy males. He used the Master's Step Test, which does not require any complicated equipment. This test was devised by Dr. Arthur M. Master in 1925. Though it's been in clinical use for almost fifty years, its use has only recently become widely accepted. It involves walking up and down two steps, turning, and walking up and down again. The test has a limited usefulness because it's difficult to go faster and faster and to get the heart rate up to 85 percent of maximal capacity.

Dr. Bellet found that ninety-five men of the 795 he tested had abnormal responses. Now we get to the important point: Within the next three years, twenty-three of these 795 men developed symptoms of coronary artery disease; sixteen of these had acute myocardial infarction, five had angina pectoris, and two died of acute heart attacks. Not all twenty-three of these men had had abnormal stress-test results, but 13 or 13.7 percent of them did. Perhaps, had they been tested on a treadmill or bicycle ergometer, many more of them would have shown positive results. Only 1.4 percent of the men with negative tests got heart attacks. In the *American Journal of Cardiology*, Dr. Bellet wrote, "The incidence of subsequent coronary heart disease was nearly ten times greater in the group with positive tests."

In a much larger study, done by Dr. Myrvin H. Ellestad of Memorial Hospital Center in Long Beach, California, 544 positive tests were recorded, out of 1,716 patients aged twenty-nine to seventy-four. Over the next eight years 31 percent of the strong positives had heart attacks, as did 9 percent of patients with equivocal results. Only 2 percent of those whose tests were negative had heart attacks. Meanwhile, angina resulted in 82 percent of the patients who had positive or equivocally positive exercise-stress tests. None of the patients with negative tests developed angina.

You must be wondering how safe an exercise test is. What are your chances of having a heart attack during the test itself, as a result of putting so much strain on the heart? The answer is, the test is very safe indeed. Remember, the doctor is observing your electrocardiograph constantly. If he sees anything severely abnormal, he will immediately stop the test. Dr. Ellestad did over 4,000 tests at maximal capacity without a single incident. A survey done some years ago showed that in possibly one in every 10,000 tests there might be a death. This was a very conservative figure; the actual figure is probably much higher even than 10,000. Most doctors could test throughout all their years in practice without having such an unfortunate experience.

There is still another way of testing, called environmental

monitoring. Your doctor can have you wear a tape-recording cardiograph and just go through your normal activities—working, exercising, sleeping. The machine takes cardiographs constantly. When the tapes are returned to the laboratory they are run off very fast, at the rate of one or two minutes for every hour of recording time, with the technician or physician watching the playback. If anything turns up, the tape is slowed down to real time and the abnormality is carefully studied. I myself have gone up in a plane with a pilot who had had a heart attack, in order to watch how well he did at various levels during takeoff and landing. (Of course, we had a copilot along, in case of difficulty.)

The great advantage of environmental testing is that the test is run over a long period of time, unlike the other tests I've described, which only take about half an hour. Under certain circumstances an individual might develop a heart irregularity over a longer period of observation. A person who dislikes his working conditions and has many problems at the office may experience rapid pulse rates under the emotional stress generated by the unpleasant situation.

Dr. Hellerstein's work on the heart's reaction during sexual intercourse was done by this method. In this way very accurate results were obtained without the need for an observer. I don't have to point out that an observer would have embarrassed the patients and resulted in a completely artificial situation.

Exercise testing is just beginning to be used as a routine examination in a few school systems. I'm glad to be able to say that more and more young students in high school and college are being tested for physical fitness. Unfortunately, a high percentage of them are in very poor physical condition. At Loma Linda University (in California) it was found that the students tested worse than most of the faculty. These days we're even beginning to test children. Dr. Jack Wilmore, at the University of California, tested boys aged eight to twelve and found some who had high cholesterol and fat levels, were obese, and were already showing abnormalities on their electrocardiographs.

The trend today seems to be toward less and less exercise, and, as a result, very poor physical fitness. College students who are not actually members of a team tend to get little or no active exercise. By the time they have graduated and taken on jobs and families they do very little outside of mowing the lawn or shoveling snow, and even this becomes dangerous for some people. This state of affairs is not a purely American phenomenon. In a survey taken in Denmark it was found that many forty-year-old women could outperform teenage girls. The women did a good deal of heavy housework and rode bicycles, while the younger women were in the habit of riding on motor bikes or in cars and spent much of their time studying. The habits of very young children have changed radically in the past few years, with the changeover to sitting on a school bus; these same youngsters' parents often walked long distances to and from school. Even the physical-education programs in the schools have changed, with increasing emphasis on teams, at the expense of the less well coordinated boys and girls, who need regular exercise for good physical condition even though they will never be star performers.

It's my hope that I've succeeded in convincing you of the importance of a regular exercise program. Its importance, in my opinion, is second only to giving up smoking as a preventative measure to cut down the risk of heart attack. But please don't embark on any form of exercise that is new to you without first going for an exercise stress test. Too much exercise, or the wrong kind of exercise, is as bad as—if not worse than—none at all.

13

Exercising—The Whys and Hows of Exercising

THE ATHLETES WHO COMPETED in the 1970 Olympic marathon ran more than 26 miles at a fast trot. The winner finished in two hours and fifteen minutes. To the hundreds of thousands of Americans who watched the Olympics from an easy chair in front of a television set, the endurance of marathon runners appears incredible.

There is no television in the mountains of northern Mexico, so we don't know how modern marathon runners might impress the Tarahumara Indians who live there. Probably not much. The Tarahumara begin to run as soon as they learn to walk. Running is their principal means of livelihood. They often hire themselves out as human moving vans because they can run farther and faster than their main competition—donkeys. The Tarahumara hunt some animals by chasing them for days until the quarry drop from exhaustion. Running is also their main sport. Not long ago a medical observer clocked eight Tarahumara men between the ages of eighteen and forty-eight during a 28-mile kickball race over craggy terrain. Including time spent looking for balls kicked off course, the winning team finished the race in four hours and forty-five minutes—an average speed of 5.8 miles per hour.

Deaths from cardiac disease or circulatory problems are unknown among the Tarahumara.

136

I mention the Tarahumara only as an example of the kind of physical activity the human body is capable of—the kind of activity, indeed, for which nature designed it. No serious physician expects modern, sedentary Americans to revert to an aboriginal life style. Civilized life, after all, does include a few pleasures other than running, even a few goals other than the avoidance of heart disease. Nor is it necessary for Americans to run for hours each day. Careful laboratory studies of the physiology of exercise have shown that you can gain substantial improvement of heart function with only one half-hour workout every other day. But the workout must consist of the right kind of physical training.

There are three possible results of physical training: an increase in the size and strength of the skeletal muscles; increased agility or the development of specific skills; and increased physical endurance. The same exercise can bring more than one desirable result; basketball, for example, increases both agility and endurance.

As far as the heart is concerned, however, endurance is the only result that counts. Unfortunately, many extremely active people, including many people in planned exercise programs, fool themselves into the mistaken belief that they are doing their hearts some good when they are merely building other muscles or becoming proficient at a sport.

Muscle-building exercises, such as weight-lifting or isometrics (tensing one muscle against another), are advisable only for those too feeble to accomplish their ordinary daily tasks. The weight lifter winds up with biceps like bowling balls and legs like beer kegs. Smeared with oil and dressed in a loin cloth, he's an ornament on any beach. Most people who need such physiques for their daily activities develop them naturally enough by engaging in the very activities that create the need. No man who spends eight hours a day digging ditches need lift weights to develop his muscles; digging ditches does the job alone and builds endurance to boot.

Weight-lifting and isometrics do little to build endurance and therefore do little for the heart. In fact, exercises such as weight-lifting may even be detrimental to the heart. Watch a weight lifter and you will observe a demonstration of the Valsalva phenomenon, so called after an eighteenth-century Italian scientist who first noticed it. As the weight lifter strains against the weight, he closes his glottis, the air passageway in the throat, to gain power. With the glottis forced shut, air pressure in his chest increases, preventing blood from returning to the heart. His veins bulge because blood has backed into them (the expression "burst a blood vessel" is rooted in accurate observation of a man working too hard at lifting or carrying). His blood pressure at first rises very rapidly, as it usually does during sudden heavy exercise. But then it falls because of the decreased blood flow to the heart. That's dangerous; strain that abnormally lowers blood pressure courts a cardiac incident. One sign of beneficial exercise is deep, rhythmical breathing, quite the reverse of the strain involved in weight lifting.

Exercises that promote agility or sharpen particular physical skills don't usually present the danger of specific muscle-building exercises. Bowling and golf are among the most popular skill-building activities. The bowler practices and practices, frame after frame, year after year, trying to boost his average to the magic 200 mark. The golfer pursues his goal weekend upon weekend, correcting hooks and slices, working on his putting game, aiming, depending on his ambition, to break 100, or 90, or (please, God!) 80.

The end result of such practice may well be a handsome trophy. But rarely is it endurance training. The bowler who bowls his two frames and then sits down to wait for his partner's turn may be having a nice time, but he's not exercising his heart. Furthermore, the better he gets, the more strikes he bowls—and the less he exerts himself. The golfer who takes his swing and then chases after the ball in an electric cart is probably getting even less real exercise than the bowler. If you bowl, or golf, or play pitty-pat on the tennis court during a weekend set of mixed doubles, by all means stick with it. Such relaxation helps cope with stress and therefore is of real benefit. But don't confuse those activities with the exercise needed to train the heart.

The only exercise result that counts so far as the heart is concerned is increased physical endurance. Simply defined, endurance is the body's ability to meet a relatively high demand for oxygen sustained for longer than a few minutes. The cells use both oxygen and food to produce energy, and blood supplies both. The cells can also store food, in the form of a substance called glycogen, against shortages in the supply of blood. But cells cannot store oxygen for more than three or four minutes. In the absence of an adequate regular oxygen supply, the cells can oxidize stored glycogen for a few minutes to produce energy—but then only at a great price in function, as we shall see later. Thus oxygen supply is a limiting factor in all physical activity.

You build muscles by forcing them to work hard; you develop skills by practicing. In the same way, you increase physical endurance by forcing your body to use large quantities of oxygen for relatively long periods of time. Endurance exercises are those that require you to move rapidly and continuously for at least fifteen minutes without stopping, so that your pulse (a rough measure of oxygen delivery) rises far above its resting rate and then remains steady at a fairly high exercise rate. The best endurance exercises are walking, running, jumping, bicycle riding, and swimming—as well as sports that require you to engage in one of those exercises continuously for fifteen minutes or more.

Endurance and endurance training are words with a tough ring to them. Yet it's surprisingly easy to build a safe and effective endurance training program into your daily schedule. Here's how to start: Put down this book, get up out of your chair, go outside, and take a walk. Walk briskly, as if marching in a parade, for fifteen minutes.

Is it cold out? Dress warmly.

Too hot? Hold off until the cool of evening, or take your walk first thing in the morning, before breakfast.

Raining? Wear rubbers and carry an umbrella.

If you don't like walking in the rain, drive to a shopping mall, park your car, and take your walk there.

However, if there's some reason why it's better not to leave the house at all—a hurricane is raging outside, or you fear there are muggers prowling the neighborhood—just march around your home for fifteen minutes. Go from room to room. If there are stairs, climb them. Beware of stray toys; ignore jeering children; and tell your spouse you will explain everything later.

As soon as the fifteen minutes are up, take your pulse. The easiest places to find a pulse are on the inside of the wrist about an inch and a half south of the thumb, and on the sides of the neck. You will need a watch with a second hand. Put a finger on the pulse, count the number of beats in ten seconds, and multiply the result by six. That's your pulse rate—the same as the number of heartbeats per minute. (Don't try to count your pulse for a full minute, because your heart will be beating more slowly at the end of the minute than it was at the start, immediately after the walk. The pulse rate you want to find is the rate during the exercise, not at some point thirty, forty, or sixty seconds later.)

Now turn to the chart on page 150. Find your age group at the left of the chart. Move your finger to the right, into the area called the Warm-up Zone. Your pulse rate immediately after the fifteen-minute walk should be in the Warm-up Zone.

Thus, if you are forty-two years old, your objective is a walk brisk enough to raise your pulse rate to between 108 and 118. If your pulse is below 108, then you have probably taken a languid stroll instead of a brisk walk. Next time, get the lead out. If your pulse is above 118, you have walked a bit too fast, or perhaps your route was uphill. Either way, take it a little easier next time. Your goal is a comfortable pace that puts your pulse rate in the Warm-up Zone for your age and keeps it there during the walk.

Tomorrow morning, as soon as you wake up and before you get out of bed, take your pulse again. That's your resting pulse, probably somewhere between 60 and 80 beats per minute. Write it down; you'll look back on it with interest several months from now.

Next step: Figure out how to fit a fifteen-minute walk into your normal daily schedule. Perhaps you can park your car half a mile to a mile from the office and walk the rest of the way. (That means a walk back after work, too, of course; so much the better.) Or maybe there's an errand you have in mind that you can do on foot instead of by car. See if your wife or husband will join you for a walk before breakfast or dinner, or in the early evening. Try walking the children to school. They may have to run to keep up, but that's more fun than the school bus and a lot healthier. Or just walk for the sake of walking.

Do it every day for two weeks, making sure your pulse rate gets into the Warm-up Zone and stays there. To make the walk a little more interesting, try hitting a pulse-rate target. Say your pulse tomorrow is exactly 110 after the walk. See if you can hit 110 on the nose again the next day. Then try for 95 the day after by slowing down just a little. Next, speed up a bit and shoot for 106. By the end of two weeks you can become pretty expert at regulating your heart rate by making small adjustments in walking pace. Learning to regulate your pulse rate will come in handy later on.

This warm-up phase of the exercise program is not endurance training. It's preparation. The stretch of mild activity is needed to accustom muscles, tendons, and joints to exercise, to help ward off the aches and pains familiar to anyone who has ever tried strenuous physical activity after a long period of doing nothing much. The warm-up period also serves as a test to make sure you can exercise comfortably—a kind of double check on your doctor's O.K. It will make you familiar with the way your heart, as measured by pulse rate, responds to mild activity. Finally, the two-week warm-up period lets you establish the *habit* of exercise by fitting the walk into your daily schedule.

After two weeks, consult the chart again for the exercise Target Zone corresponding to your age. If you're between forty and forty-four years old, for example, the Target Zone is a pulse rate of between 128 and 154 beats per minute. Endurance training takes place when, and only when, you get your pulse up into that Target Zone and keep it there for between fifteen and twenty minutes.

Now that you have a pulse target, choose a basic endurance activity with which to hit it. Pick an exercise that you can conveniently do every other day. If you live in Florida, or California, or Arizona, and if you have a pool in the backyard, you might want to make swimming the basic activity. If there's little traffic in your neighborhood, perhaps you can count on bicycling every other day. If you prefer indoor activity, consider a stationary exercise bicycle. Hedonists can pedal away while watching television, intellectuals while reading a book.

For most people, though, the most versatile, convenient, and inexpensive basic exercise is locomotion—a word I use to cover the simple, natural act of going from here to there on foot. That exercise includes walking (slow locomotion), jogging (medium-speed locomotion), and running (fast locomotion). You can locomote anywhere—suburban roads, beaches, cinder tracks, city streets, up and down stairways. You can locomote at home, from one room to another or in place, or at the office. Locomotion requires no expensive equipment. You can locomote in your usual clothing if you don't want people to know what you're doing, or in a track suit if you do. Finally, locomotion is a part of almost every active game—tennis, touch football, basketball, handball, golf—so you can easily substitute a supporting activity for the basic locomotion whenever you get a chance.

What kind of locomotion is best? That's between you and your pulse rate. Young people will probably find that they have to run to get their pulse rate into the Target Zone; elderly people will discover that a walk does the trick. Furthermore, the kind of locomotion will change with your physical condition. Again, your pulse rate will tell you when and how. A fifty-year-old man who reaches his Target Zone by walking may discover after a month or so that walking no longer suffices. He can't walk fast enough to get his pulse above 120, the start of his Target Zone. He must break into a jog to do it. That's a good sign. It shows that his heart is working more efficiently, since it supplies the oxygen demanded by walking with fewer beats per minute than previously.

When you've settled on a basic activity, set aside half an hour for a full exercise cycle—five to ten minutes in the Warm-up Zone, fifteen to twenty minutes in the Target Zone, and another five minutes of activity back in the Warm-up Zone.

To start off, push your pulse into the Warm-up Zone with a couple of minutes of slow locomotion; by now you should have the right pace down cold. Or you can warm up with calisthenics—knee bends, toe touches, push-ups, and the like. Calisthenics are especially good for those who want to strengthen particular groups of muscles. Sit-ups, for example, strengthen the abdominal muscles and help prevent middle-age paunch. If you can't touch your toes or keep your back straight during a push-up, don't strain. After a few weeks of calisthenic warm-up, stiff muscles will grow more elastic and weak muscles will grow stronger. Meanwhile, concentrate on pushing your pulse rate into the Warm-up Zone. Keep it there for two or three minutes, then gradually work a little faster so that the pulse moves toward the Target Zone. After five to ten minutes (five minutes for thirty-year-olds, ten minutes for sixty-year-olds), break into the basic Target Zone activity or a substitute.

Don't skip the warm-up to save time. It's called a warm-up because light exercise raises the temperature of the muscles. That helps to loosen up muscles and joints, making sprains and strains during the Target Zone activity less likely. The warm-up also opens the capillary network in the muscles (including the heart muscle) in preparation for an increased flow of blood, so there's less chance of the kind of temporary oxygen shortage that sudden vigorous activity can produce.

Next comes the Target Zone activity. If your basic activity is locomotion, take off at a pace slightly faster than the pace that put you in the Warm-up Zone. For a man or woman of forty, the Target Zone locomotion might be an easy jog, for the sixty-year-old, perhaps a fast walk. After a minute or two, stop and check your pulse. If it's not in the Target Zone, locomote a little faster. Check again after another minute. If your pulse goes above the Target Zone, slow down. By trial and error you'll soon find the locomotion pace that regulates your pulse in the middle of the Target Zone.

The same principle of letting your pulse rate control the activity applies to all endurance exercises. Swimmers can check at the end of each lap; bicyclists when stopped at a crossroad. Once you get the feel of your own body's response to various levels of exercise, you won't have to stop very often.

Whenever you increase your level of physical activity— when you rise from a chair to walk to the television set, when you move from a stroll to a fast walk or from a fast walk to a jog—your muscles and other organs demand more oxygen than you have been taking in. You breathe a little faster and deeper to take in more oxygen, your heart beats a little faster to move the oxygen to the demanding cells, and all the mechanisms that make for efficient use of oxygen come into play.

Thus, oxygen demand and supply come into balance almost automatically. If you continue your new level of activity you will reach what is called a *steady state*. Pulse rate is the indicator of the steady state. In the transition from Warm-up Zone to Target Zone activity, your pulse may rise from, say, 110 to 140. But at some point soon after you settle down to a steady pace—a jog, for example—your pulse rate will stop rising, and level off at some high plateau. That's the signal that oxygen demand and supply have reached a new balance. In theory, you can continue a steady-state activity indefinitely; you will never run out of oxygen. It is because they reach a steady state at a high level of oxygen demand that the Tarahumara can run for hour after hour, mile after mile. (In practice, however, skeletal muscles do tire out for reasons other than a shortage of oxygen, so don't try for marathon distances without professional training.)

If after reaching a steady state you increase the pace again —from a jog to a run, for example—you again increase oxygen demand. Up goes the respiration rate and up goes the heart rate in search of a new balance. At some level of activity, however, the body will be unable to reach a balance between oxygen supply and demand. You risk approaching that level of activity when your pulse rate rises into the area of the chart called the Danger Zone.

If you have passed a physical examination and exercise test and have finished the thirty-day warm-up period without discomfort, you can be reasonably well assured that you will reach a comfortable and safe steady state at pulse rates within the Target Zone for your age. Most people will also find comfortable steady states in the Danger Zone. *But there is no advantage to be gained from exercise at that level, and there is good reason to avoid it.*

At some point in the Danger Zone the body goes into a condition of oxygen debt—the muscles use more oxygen than the circulatory system can deliver. The debt must be repaid by slowing down, or you will collapse. The combination of oxygen and glycogen that produces energy also leaves waste products in the form of carbon dioxide and lactic acid. The blood carries those waste products from the cells after delivering oxygen. The carbon dioxide is carried to the lungs and is exhaled. The lactic acid is carried to the liver, where most of it is processed for excretion through the urine.

Even under the best circumstances of oxygen balance, however, some lactic acid remains in muscle cells. It is the slow accumulation of lactic acid that results in muscular fatigue; in fact, lactic acid is called "the acid of fatigue." It is the slow build-up of lactic acid in the leg muscles, not any weakness of the heart muscle or any danger of heart failure, that finally puts a limit on how far a marathon runner can run. Eventually lactic acid builds to the point where a runner's legs collapse under him or her. It is because of a slow accumulation of lactic acid that you feel tired at the end of the day. During sleep, with muscular activity at a minimum, most of the lactic acid is removed from the muscle cells and you awake refreshed in the morning. Although they probably don't know it, it is to allow the lactic-acid level to decline that fighters rest the day before a fight rather than continue training and that football teams take their last heavy practice on the Thursday before a Saturday game rather than on Friday.

Under the condition of oxygen debt that results from prolonged activity in the Danger Zone, however, lactic acid builds up rapidly rather than slowly. The result is best illustrated by describing what happens to a miler out to break a world's record. He starts off at the fastest clip he can comfortably maintain. By the end of the first lap he has probably reached a steady state at a fairly high pulse rate; he's spending great amounts of energy but taking in and distributing enough oxygen to meet the demand. Then, at some point in the last lap he pulls out the stops and runs as fast as he possibly can. His pulse rate rises rapidly as his heart tries to meet the enormous demand for oxygen imposed by the effort, but his pulse is now well up in the Danger Zone and continuing to rise. With his body in a condition of oxygen debt, lactic acid quickly accumulates in the leg muscles. If the runner times his effort perfectly, he will collapse just as he reaches the tape, having pushed himself to exhaustion. Prone, he will gasp for breath and gulp air hungrily, seeking to repay part of the oxygen debt. After a small repayment he will be helped to his feet and walk on partially recovered legs, breathing deeply and repaying the rest of the debt.

Your Danger Zone, as shown on the chart, is the zone in which you will incur a similar debt. The danger may not be primarily to your heart, but to injury due to falls that may result from lactic-acid fatigue. But there is a possibility of heart damage in the Danger Zone. Remember, your physical examination pronounced you fit for physical activity up to the level at which you were tested. That level should have been above that of the Target Zone. But you were not tested to maximal exertion, so there is no way of telling whether or when extremely high levels of exertion will result in dangerous shortages in the heart's oxygen supply. It's best not to allow your pulse to go into the Danger Zone for any extended period of time.

That doesn't mean you must shun the low edge of the Danger Zone as a bather would shun shark-infested waters. A particularly hard rally in tennis, one that sends you up to the net and back to the baseline and then from one corner to the other at top speed, might push your pulse rate into the Danger Zone briefly. But the short pause between the end of the point and the next service will bring the pulse (and the oxygen demand) down before there's much chance of a damaging shortage. Test yourself. If your pulse rate is in the Danger Zone, slow down.

During your first few basic exercise periods, check your pulse whenever you feel a decided change in respiration. If you start to breathe very hard, it's a sign that your body may be demanding too much oxygen. Make sure your pulse isn't in the Danger Zone. By the same token, if breathing becomes very easy you may not be working hard enough. Again, your pulse rate will tell the story. Before long you will know just how fast you need to locomote, or pedal a bike, or swim, or jump a rope to keep the pulse rate in the Target Zone.

Distance doesn't matter much. If two forty-year-old walkers locomote for fifteen minutes, both moving fast enough to maintain a pulse rate of 140, one may cover a mile in fifteen minutes and the other a mile and one-quarter. But their stimulus for endurance training has been nearly equal. Nor does speed matter much, since two people of the same age may well have to move at different speeds to maintain identical pulse rates.

Duration matters only up to a point. For most people, the physical changes that result in the efficient use of oxygen just don't take place unless the pulse rate stays in the Target Zone for at least fifteen minutes. According to Dr. Sam Fox of Georgetown University School of Medicine you need at least fifteen minutes, three times a week.

Target Zone activity that lasts longer than twenty minutes, however, doesn't necessarily result in proportional improvement in endurance. That is, you don't double the benefits to your body by doubling to thirty or forty minutes the time you spend in the Target Zone. Fifteen to twenty minutes of Target Zone activity will result in a substantial training effect. A lot more time brings only a little additional improvement. If you want to exercise for more than twenty minutes, you'll probably want to take up a substitute activity and spend the extra time practicing specific skills.

Almost any physical activity you enjoy can become a substitute for the basic activity. Take golf as an example. Next time you play, don't rent a cart. Locomote to your ball, take your swing, and start locomoting again. At the third tee, check your pulse. If you're in the Target Zone, fine. Keep playing that way. If not, locomote faster—trot after the ball. When you learn to play golf in your Target Zone, you have a substitute activity.

The same principle applies to tennis. Check your pulse every other game, when you change courts. Chances are it will be in the Target Zone during a set of singles. If it's a little shy, move a bit more. Skip from side to side while awaiting service, the way the pros do. Go after balls you would normally let pass. Rush the net more frequently. That should get your pulse into the Target Zone—and it may even improve your game. There's another target activity.

Come leaf-raking time in the fall, try raking as if you were being paid by the job rather than by the hour. If you work fast enough you can get that pulse rate up. Then you can substitute fifteen to twenty minutes of leaf-raking for the basic activity. Other types of work around the house—sawing wood, turning soil for a vegetable garden, shoveling snow—are potential substitute activities. Just monitor the pulse rate. (The mention of snow-shoveling no doubt brings to mind the perennial wintertime news stories of men dropping dead while shoveling snow. If you have spent a month of daily activity in the Warm-up Zone, if you warm up before picking up the shovel, and if you make sure to shovel at a pace that keeps your pulse in the Target Zone, you're safer shoveling snow than driving in it.)

What happens if you exercise less frequently than every other day? If you exercise much less frequently, say only once or twice a week, the training effect may not take place. If you have already gotten into shape, you will predictably fall out of shape in a matter of weeks if you exercise but once a week. Still, there is no need to attack your exercise program compulsively. If you don't feel well, don't exercise. If circumstances force you to cancel today's half hour, fit it in tomorrow. And if you miss a whole week, start again slowly by staying in the Warm-up Zone for the full half hour over the next couple of weeks.

Always finish your exercise period with five or ten minutes of the basic activity at a gradually diminishing pace or with appropriate walking. During the Target Zone activity the heart has pushed out blood rapidly to meet the demand, and the flexing and unflexing of muscles in the arms and legs has helped squeeze the blood through the veins back to the heart just as rapidly. If you stop cold your heart will continue to beat rapidly for a while. But with the muscles no longer contracting, there's nothing to help the veins move the blood back to the heart from the extremities. Blood may then pool in the legs, resulting in a shortage of oxygen to the brain and possible faintness or dizziness. Five minutes of mild activity after the Target Zone exercise keeps the blood circulating while the heart gradually slows down.

If you shower just after the activity, make the water tepid, not hot. Hot water opens the blood vessels, with the potential of aggravating any tendency for blood to pool. Stay away from saunas and steam baths until you've cooled off.

After you have been on Target Zone activity for two months, take your pulse again before you get out of bed in the morning. Compare your new resting pulse rate with the resting rate you wrote down at the start of the exercise program. It's probably significantly lower—a dramatic sign of increased heart efficiency.

PULSE RATES DURING EXERCISE

AGE	WARM-UP ZONE	TARGET ZONE	DANGER ? ZONE	MAXIMAL PULSE
30-34	116-126	136-164	Above 164	194
35-39	112-122	132-160	Above 160	188
40-44	108-118	128-154	Above 154	182
45-49	104-114	124-150	Above 150	176
50-54	100-110	120-146	Above 146	170
55-59	96-106	116-140	Above 140	166
60-64	92-102	112-136	Above 136	160
65 and over	86- 96	106-130	Above 130	154

14

How to Find Out About Yourself – The Odds

THROUGHOUT THIS BOOK I've been talking about hearts. Now it's time to talk about you. Will *you* beat the odds on a heart attack? Nobody can tell you that for sure, not even your doctor. But together you and he can make a pretty fair guess—a guess good enough to act on.

On pages 152–153 is a questionnaire. Fill it out and you can score your own chances. There's a trick to the questionnaire, though—you can't fill it out alone. You can do it only with the help of the physical examination and laboratory tests provided by a physician. So the place to start figuring your odds is in your doctor's office.

Don't feel shy about asking the doctor for the precise results of the tests. What are the blood-pressure numbers? What exactly are your serum cholesterol and triglyceride figures? What does the glucose-tolerance test show? Are you physically fit? It's your body; you have a right to the answers. The answers are easy enough for the doctor to get through routine tests that a physician should do during the course of a thorough examination.

A questionnaire which is called *Risko* and was developed by the Michigan Heart Association is similar to the one you're answering and was returned by 654 persons in a study in New Jersey. Of these, sixty-seven persons (10 percent) had scores

WILL YOU BEAT THE ODDS?

Circle the box that best describes your condition, in each case.

1. WEIGHT (If your weight at the age of 25 was satisfactory, use that figure for your ideal weight.)

   Lean   1 point   Normal   2 points

                    Overweight   3 points

2. BLOOD PRESSURE (Choose the figure to which you are closest.)

   Below 130/80   1 point   140/90   2 points

                    Above 160/95   3 points

3. SMOKING

   Nonsmoker   1 point   Smoke 10 cigarettes   2 points
                                        or fewer daily

                    Smoke 20 cigarettes   3 points
                        or more daily

4. EXERCISE HABITS

   Very active   1 point   Moderately active   2 points

                    Inactive   3 points

5. SERUM CHOLESTEROL

   Below 200   1 point   200–250   2 points

                    Above 250   3 points

6. SERUM TRIGLYCERIDES (Choose the figure to which you are closest.)

   Below 150   1 point   200 or above   2 points

                    250 or above   3 points

7. GLUCOSE TOLERANCE

   Nondiabetic   1 point   Tendency to diabetes   2 points

                    Diabetes   3 points

8. EMOTIONAL STRESS

Easygoing   1 point   Moderately tense   2 points

Very nervous   3 points

9. HEREDITY (Number of parents, grandparents, brothers, and sisters under age sixty with history of heart attack or stroke.)

None   1 point   One   2 points

Two or more   3 points

10. EXERCISE STRESS TEST

Very fit   1 point   Average   2 points

Unfit   3 points

TOTAL POINTS

10 — Your chances of having a heart attack before sixty are very low.

11–16 — Not bad, but it wouldn't hurt to reexamine your habits.

17–22 — Average American and thus a poor risk.

22 + — You are in danger, and it is urgent that you see your doctor.

---

that placed them in the lowest-risk category, well below average, and ninety-one (14 percent) had scores near the top of the scale, indicating urgent danger—a need to reduce their scores immediately. The remaining 496 (76 percent) had scores indicating an average to moderate risk.

* * *

Let's say you are one of those rare persons who has a score of 10. You must be doing something right. You were probably lucky in your choice of ancestors, and right in your choice of life style. Don't change a thing. The chances of your having a

premature heart attack—an attack before you're over sixty—
is very low. If you do have a heart attack, it will probably be
in what is considered old age. People like you almost never
have heart attacks in their forties.

* * *

If your score is between 11 and 16, you have a few risk
factors going against you. You may avoid having a heart attack
for a very long time, but it wouldn't hurt you to reexamine
your habits and make whatever improvement you can. If
you're overweight or your cholesterol is too high, follow my
recommendations for lowering those scores.

* * *

If your score is between 17 and 22, you undoubtedly have
just about the same number of risk factors as most of your
friends. In other words, you are average. Unfortunately, the
average American is not a very healthy person. Over 50 percent of Americans die of heart attacks, and the majority of
those people were considered average. In another country,
your American "average" score would put you in a poor-risk
category. It's urgent that you start on a program to reduce your
risk factors. If you don't, your chances of having a heart attack
soon are too great to ignore. I suggest you reread the pertinent
chapters of this book and discuss them with your physician.

* * *

If your score is near 30, you have practically all the risk
factors going against you. You have something to worry about.
If your doctor isn't worried, find another doctor. You are in
danger. You need a doctor who recognizes the danger *before*
you have a cardiac event.

An event can be anginal chest pain, a heart attack, such as
myocardial infarction, or a heart attack so massive that it results in sudden death. Any recognizable positive symptom is an

event. Dr. Seymour Dayton puts it this way: "The event is the surfacing of obvious illness. If we can get the patient to reduce his risk factors, we may be able to keep the disease process from surfacing again. If he doesn't reduce them, the chances are high that another event will occur." Your doctor can help reduce your danger significantly both by medical means and by impressing you personally with the necessity of major changes in the way you live.

You must be wondering (and worrying) about just how much can be done for those who have increased risk factors. Dr. Jeremiah Stamler, the medical director of the Chicago Coronary Prevention Evaluation Program, did an interesting study along these lines, taking a group of 390 men who were at high risk and putting them into a preventative program. He instructed these men to go on diets (to lose weight and lower the lipid levels in their blood), to exercise sensibly, and to quit smoking. Over the next seven years only two of these men suffered fatal heart attacks.

Dr. Herman Hellerstein of Case-Western Reserve Medical College in Cleveland, a pioneer in the use of exercise as prevention against heart attack, did a nine-year study with a group of 650 cardiac-prone (high-risk) patients. He had them exercise at 60 to 70 percent of their maximum oxygen-uptake capacity three times every week for periods of one hour. Meanwhile, a control group of 350 did not participate in the program.

An impressive 80 percent of the patients on the program showed great improvement after an average of three-and a half years. Their exercise electrocardiograms were improved, and they had lower blood pressure, lower cholesterol levels, improved heart function, and better oxygen uptake. The death rate among those 650 patients was 1.9, compared to 5.0 in the controls.

This study caused Dr. Hellerstein to conclude that inducing patients to quit smoking and to eat the recommended diet, in addition to participating in an exercise program, may very well cut the death rate by two-thirds. Dr. Hellerstein is not prepared to commit himself further than this cautious "may" because the patients in his study were not carefully selected. These patients had volunteered for the program. It's possible that only the type of person who is less likely to have a heart attack chooses to participate in such a program. Those more likely to have heart trouble might not want to take part, he says.

* * *

So much for the patient who has never had an event. Let's go on to talk about those who have had one, in the form of angina. I can't give angina patients formal medical advice or prescribe any sort of therapy without a complete examination. Every case is different, and generalizations would be extremely dangerous. The only advice that is safe for me to give is this: If you haven't already done so, see your doctor and let him obtain all the necessary information about your particular problem. These days, there are many kinds of examinations that were unheard of fifteen years ago.

One of the most useful new tools we have is the angiogram. This technique involves putting a radio-opaque liquid into the coronary arteries. The liquid serves to outline the arteries. Then, when x-rays are taken, we can see precisely to what degree the arteries are obstructed by atherosclerosis. This examination is only advisable in certain cases; in others, its use is not yet considered necessary. Once again, only your own doctor can decide what tests he or she will need in order to obtain the necessary information.

Sometimes an operation on the coronary arteries is indicated, to bypass a block and restore circulation. In another case medication will do the job, with no need for surgery. In still another case, reducing the risk factors and increasing the amount and quality of exercise is enough to recondition the heart.

Dr. John E. Smith, chief of cardiovascular services for United Air Lines, put twenty-one pilots with symptoms of angina on a walking routine. He started them out walking a mile in twenty minutes, four times a day. He worked them up very gradually, until they could do that mile in nine minutes. Dr. Smith was delighted to find that fifteen of these men stopped having anginal pain and their exercise EKGs improved.

Similar results are being reported by Dr. Lenore R. Zohman of Einstein Medical College. Dr. Zohman used the bicycle exercise in a supine position for her testing. She then had her patients train for six weeks at an exercise level just below that which caused anginal pain. All eighteen of her patients reported a decrease in pain, said that they needed less nitroglycerine and were able to work better. She also found improvements in the EKGs of eight of these patients, even on this very brief program.

You'll notice that in both Dr. Smith's and Dr. Zohman's programs only some of the patients showed great improvement. Others failed to get better. That's why I must reiterate that each patient problem has a solution all its own.

* * *

Now let's go one step further, from the patient suffering from angina to the one who has had an actual heart attack with some muscle damage—myocardial infarction. What can be done? Once again, much depends on the individual case—just how much damage has been done. Some patients may need to have an operative procedure performed on their arteries, as already described, followed by a risk factor reduction program. In other cases, treatment with medications or with rehabilitation exercise programs, or both, is the best way.

If your doctor decides on a rehabilitation program, this would call for a reduction of risk factors and reconditioning routine for the heart muscle, as I've described in the chapter on exercise testing and exercise techniques. In many cases your doctor will start you on a program of gentle exercises while you're still in bed, possibly within a few days after your admission to the hospital. In cases in which the attack is more severe, your doctor will prefer to wait awhile before starting you on exercise. After you've left the hospital you may be put on a program of short walks. As you continue to improve, the walks will be lengthened, calisthenics will be added, and then participation in sports may be encouraged. Eventually—subject to close supervision by your doctor—greater effort may be advisable. Only your own physician or a knowledgeable consultant can judge what is the best procedure for your individual problem.

You have probably read something about the graduated programs already underway in some cities, and you must be wondering how successful they have been for those able to enter them. In Toronto, Dr. Peter A. Rechnitzer and his group did a detailed evaluation of 77 patients, all of whom had stayed with an exercise program for at least three months, and 111 controls. The evaluation was done over a five-year period. It showed that only 1.3 percent of the exercise group had had a nonfatal recurrence, while 27.9 percent of the controls had recurrences. There were three deaths (3.9 percent) in the exercising group, but there were fifteen deaths (11.8 percent) in the control group. Dr. Rechnitzer warns that these results must be interpreted with caution since other variables, unrelated to the exercise program, may have had some effect in these optimistic results.

Let's take a quick journey from Canada to Israel, where Dr. J. J. Kellermann runs a rehabilitation institution. He worked with a group of forty-four patients who had suffered myocardial infarction. These patients participated in an exercise program for at least a year; some of them exercised for as long as fifty-four months. Dr. Kellermann reports that of this group of patients, only three (7 percent) died of heart attacks, and five (13 percent) suffered a recurrence. Meanwhile, in a control group of ninety-two patients, twenty (22 percent) died of heart attack and nine (17 percent) had recurrences. The mean age of these patients was fifty-six years.

Dr. Kellermann also cautions against attributing too much importance to the value of the exercise program alone. He points out that the patients who had such good results came to the institute twice a week, for years, and received constant medical guidance. They were given help and encouragement in controlling their weight and diet, and equally constant *discouragement* about smoking. He stresses the value of the psychological factor involved in belonging to such a group and points out that patients with all this going for them can't be compared with other groups that don't have the benefit of such guidance along with the physical training.

So much for the conclusions of that study in Israel. Let's return to North America, this time to Boston, where each year they run a race known as the Boston Marathon. The distance covered in a marathon is 26 miles, 385 yards. No doubt you are wondering why such an odd figure is used. The distance was chosen by the British Olympic committee in 1908. They started the race, that year, from the royal residence at Windsor castle and ended it in front of the royal box at the stadium in London. I'm sure you are also wondering why I brought up the matter of the Boston Marathon in a book about heart attack. You may find this hard to believe: Eight Canadians, all of whom had had heart attacks, ran in that race, and seven finished the course! These men had trained under Dr. Terence Kavanagh, medical director of the Toronto Rehabilitation Centre.

Following their heart attacks, the men had started walking, then they began to trot, and went on to jog, all before they were able to run. As their training continued, they worked up to a matter of 50 miles each week, running at a speed of a ten-minute mile, and sometimes even an eight-minute mile. No, none of the men won the marathon, but none of them came in last, either. What's important, from our point of view, is that they made such an outstanding recovery from their myocardial infarctions and were able to expend all this effort without any ill effects.

I would like to end this book on an optimistic note. I can honestly say that things are looking up for victims of heart attack. The whole concept of the coronary-care unit is new and hopeful. These units were first established only about ten years ago. They make it possible to save lives by prompt diagnosis and treatment.

Although overall deaths from heart disease have increased in this country, the death rate in the productive years (thirty-five to sixty-four) has started to drop. Yes, the age-adjusted death rate peaked in 1963 and has since been declining, according to Dr. Peter L. Frommer, a cardiologist at the National Heart and Lung Institute. We doctors believe that this decline is due to earlier detection and better management of heart attacks.

As I have continually stressed throughout this book, even more effective than good care AFTER a heart attack is total PREVENTION of the attack. You can help yourself in the ways I have outlined—cutting out cigarettes, modifying your diet, exercising sensibly. You can start your children out on the road to better health. You can even help exert pressure on our agriculture and food industries to make the necessary changes in their present methods. I hope and believe that the day will come when most American hearts will wear out only as the result of extreme old age.